Manual of Interventional Oncology

Douglas M. Coldwell, MD, PhD, FSIR, FACR, FAHA
Professor and Vice Chair of Radiology
Professor of Bioengineering
Director, Vascular and Interventional Radiology
Department of Radiology
University of Louisville
Louisville, Kentucky

118 illustrations

Thieme
New York • Stuttgart • Delhi • Rio de Janeiro

Executive Editor: William Lamsback
Managing Editor: J. Owen Zurhellen IV
Editorial Assistant: Mary Wilson
Director, Editorial Services: Mary Jo Casey
Production Editor: Torsten Scheihagen
Editorial Director: Sue Hodgson
International Production Director:
  Andreas Schabert
International Marketing Director: Fiona Henderson
International Sales Director: Louisa Turrell
Director of Institutional Sales: Adam Bernacki
Senior Vice President and Chief Operating Officer:
  Sarah Vanderbilt
President: Brian D. Scanlan
Printer: Everbest Printing Co.

Library of Congress Cataloging-in-Publication Data

Names: Coldwell, Douglas M., author.
Title: Manual of interventional radiology /
  Douglas M. Coldwell.
Description: First edition. | New York : Thieme,
  [2018] | Includes bibliographical references and
  index.
Identifiers: LCCN 2017027466 (print) | LCCN
  2017028067 (ebook) | ISBN 9781626231962
  (E-book) | ISBN 9781626231382 (pbk. : alk. paper)
  | ISBN 9781626231962 (ebook)
Subjects: | MESH: Neoplasms--radiotherapy | Combined
  Modality Therapy--methods | Radiology,
  Interventional--organization & administration |
  Radiology, Interventional--methods
Classification: LCC RC271.R3 (ebook) | LCC RC271.R3
  (print) | NLM QZ 269 | DDC 616.99/4064--dc23
LC record available at https://lccn.loc.gov/2017027466

Important note: Medicine is an ever-changing science undergoing continual development. Research and clinical experience are continually expanding our knowledge, in particular our knowledge of proper treatment and drug therapy. Insofar as this book mentions any dosage or application, readers may rest assured that the authors, editors, and publishers have made every effort to ensure that such references are in accordance with **the state of knowledge at the time of production of the book.**

Nevertheless, this does not involve, imply, or express any guarantee or responsibility on the part of the publishers in respect to any dosage instructions and forms of applications stated in the book. **Every user is requested to examine carefully** the manufacturers' leaflets accompanying each drug and to check, if necessary in consultation with a physician or specialist, whether the dosage schedules mentioned therein or the contraindications stated by the manufacturers differ from the statements made in the present book. Such examination is particularly important with drugs that are either rarely used or have been newly released on the market. Every dosage schedule or every form of application used is entirely at the user's own risk and responsibility. The authors and publishers request every user to report to the publishers any discrepancies or inaccuracies noticed. If errors in this work are found after publication, errata will be posted at www.thieme.com on the product description page.

Some of the product names, patents, and registered designs referred to in this book are in fact registered trademarks or proprietary names even though specific reference to this fact is not always made in the text. Therefore, the appearance of a name without designation as proprietary is not to be construed as a representation by the publisher that it is in the public domain.

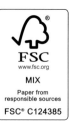

FSC
www.fsc.org
MIX
Paper from
responsible sources
FSC® C124385

Cover design: Thieme Publishing Group
Typesetting by DiTech Process Solutions

Printed in China by Everbest Printing Co. 5 4 3 2 1

ISBN 978-1-62623-138-2

Also available as an e-book:
eISBN 978-1-62623-196-2

I dedicate this book to my wife, Jane, who motivated, harassed, and helped me in so many ways to get this work completed. Without her help, this book could not have been realized.

Contents

Preface ix

Acknowledgments ix

Contributors xi

1 Essentials of Medical Oncology 1
   Vivek R. Sharma

2 Essentials of Surgical Oncology 10
   Robert C. G. Martin II

3 Essentials of Radiation Oncology 16
   Andrew S. Kennedy

4 Interventional Radiology in the
   Treatment of the Cancer Patient 33
   Douglas M. Coldwell

5 Chemotherapeutic Agents 88
   Douglas M. Coldwell

6 Colorectal Cancer 104
   Douglas M. Coldwell

7 Cancer of the Pancreas 113
   Douglas M. Coldwell

8 Carcinoid Tumor
   (Neuroendocrine Tumors of the Gastrointestinal Tract) 122
   Douglas M. Coldwell

9 Hepatocellular Carcinoma 126
   Douglas M. Coldwell

10 Cholangiocarcinoma 132
   Douglas M. Coldwell

11 Lung Cancer (Non–Small Cell) 144
   Douglas M. Coldwell

12 Head and Neck Cancer 154
   Douglas M. Coldwell

13 Renal Cell Carcinoma 161
   Douglas M. Coldwell

14 Urothelial Cancer and Transitional Cell Cancer 168
   Douglas M. Coldwell

15 Prostate Cancer 175
   Douglas M. Coldwell

16 Breast Cancer 185
   Douglas M. Coldwell

17 Gynecologic Tumors 191
   Douglas M. Coldwell

18 Clinical Trials and Interventional Oncology 199
   Douglas M. Coldwell

19 Building an Interventional Oncology Practice 206
   Douglas M. Coldwell

Index 211

Preface

Writing this book on minimally invasive, image-guided approaches to the treatment of solid tumors has been the culmination of over 30 years of training, reading, practice, more reading, and learning from all oncologic healthcare providers with whom I have worked. No interventional radiologist has the credentials currently to refer to themselves as an interventional oncologist without significant study over and above their training in fellowship. Without gaining insight into the approaches other cancer specialties utilize to treat the cancer patient and understanding what their strengths and weaknesses are, we can't have a good understanding of where we fit into the broader scheme of things. I hope this book will aid in making the transition.

An overview of the "traditional" oncologic specialties—surgery, medical, and radiation—is given first, followed by the essential procedures used in the treatment of cancer patients. A review of commonly used chemotherapy agents at the time of this writing is presented, followed by synopses of specific tumors in which IO has had an impact. Each tumor's pathology, epidemiology, genetics, staging, treatment, outcomes, and potentials for IO is given. Finally, a road map to developing an IO practice is outlined. I have utilized this plan successfully over the years.

Thanks to my contributors, this book is a cross-section of the treatments available and when and how they are utilized. I encourage all who read this book to go on to learn more about oncology and advance our field of interventional oncology.

Acknowledgments

I want to especially recognize the role my mentor, Sidney Wallace, had in motivating me to accept interventional oncology as a calling. We all have "professional DNA" and I am proud to say that Sidney was my most influential progenitor.

I also want to express my gratitude to all those medical, surgical, and radiation oncologists from whom I have learned so much, especially those three who have taken the time and made the effort to contribute to this work.

Finally, my family, friends, residents, colleagues, and, most of all, patients, have encouraged me during the writing process, and so they deserve my deepest gratitude and sincere appreciation.

Contributors

Douglas M. Coldwell, MD, PhD, FSIR, FACR, FAHA
Professor and Vice Chair of Radiology
Professor of Bioengineering
Director, Vascular and Interventional Radiology
Department of Radiology
University of Louisville
Louisville, Kentucky

Andrew S. Kennedy, MD, FACRO
Director, Radiation Oncology Research
Sarah Cannon Research Institute
Nashville, Tennessee

Robert C. G. Martin II, MD, PhD
Professor of Surgery
Director, Surgical Oncology
University of Louisville
Louisville, Kentucky

Vivek R. Sharma, MD, FACP
Associate Professor of Medicine
Division of Medicine Oncology/Hematology
University of Louisville
Louisville, Kentucky

1 Essentials of Medical Oncology

Vivek R. Sharma

Introduction

The purpose of this chapter is to give the reader an in-depth understanding of the overarching principles that guide the current practice of medical oncology and its role in the management of the cancer patient. It is not intended to provide details about individual drugs or the management of any one particular type of cancer but rather to serve as a general overview that complements the reviews on the roles of surgical and radiation oncology.

In the simplest of terms, the specialty of medical oncology involves the use of systemic therapy in the treatment of cancer. This would be the ideal way to treat the disease if we had highly effective and minimally toxic agents such as we do for example for treating various infectious diseases. However, that is presently not the case in oncology where most available agents, even though active, are often not curative. Further, most of these have significant toxicities that require them to be administered with substantial caution and close monitoring. The following sections will review the general principles of how they are used by themselves as well as in combination with other anti-cancer modalities to maximize therapeutic benefits and minimize toxicities.

Historical Background

The term "systemic therapy" implies administration of a chemical or biological agent in such a way that it enters the blood stream and distributes through the entire body to produce its therapeutic effect. Although this approach has been used in some form or fashion since ancient times, the modern era of chemotherapy began in the 1940s with the demonstration that nitrogen mustard, a derivative of mustard gas that was used as a chemical weapon during the first world war and was found to cause severe lymphoid and myeloid depletion in its victims, had therapeutic activity in lymphoma.[1] Subsequent advancement in the field was rather sporadic over the next several decades with more agents such as methotrexate being developed that showed impressive activity in hematological malignancies and even led to cure in choriocarcinoma.[2] However, optimism remained low as benefits were typically transient and toxicities were not trivial.

A significant turning point came in the mid-1960s when Drs. Holland, Freireich, and Frei used a combination of chemotherapeutic agents to cure patients with leukemia and this strategy was subsequently used by other investigators to cure lymphomas and testicular cancer.[3,4,5,6,7,8,9] The number and types of available agents have since increased, but the idea of using combinations to achieve the best outcomes still remains the predominant therapeutic approach used by medical oncologists. In the 1990s, monoclonal antibodies were introduced for the treatment of cancer with rituximab for non-Hodgkin lymphoma and trastuzumab for breast cancer.[10,11,12,13] Several others have since been added for various cancers (**Table 1.1**). Also, small molecule tyrosine kinase inhibitors were introduced in the late 1990s in the form of Bcr/Abl antagonist, imatinib mesylate for treatment of chronic myeloid leukemia.[14,15] This strategy has been subsequently applied to several other targets in various tumor types (**Table 1.2**). Other novel approaches that appear promising include agents that modulate the immune system to target cancer cells. Among these are monoclonal antibodies that block the immune check points cytotoxic T-lymphocyte-associated protein 4 (CTLA-4; Ipilimumab) or programmed death 1 (PD-1; Nivolumab, Pembrolizumab) on immune cells. They were initially tested and Food and Drug Association (FDA) approved for treatment of malignant melanoma but have since showed activity in several other tumor types.[16,17] Additional immunotherapeutic strategies include oncolytic viruses (Talimogene laherparepvec [T-VEC]) that disrupt cancer cells and trigger an immune response against them[18] and the use of adaptive immunity by way of genetically engineered T-cells (chimeric antigen receptor T cell [CART]).[19]

Table 1.1 Examples of therapeutic monoclonal antibodies in oncology

Monoclonal antibodies	Targets	Malignancies
• Trastuzumab	Her2 neu	Breast, gastric/esophageal
• Rituximab	CD20	Lymphoma, leukemia
• Bevacizumab	VEGF	Colon, lung (adeno), ovarian, cervical, GBM
• Cetuximab	EGFR	Colon, squamous cell head and neck
• Ipilumimab	CTLA-4	Melanoma
• Pembrolizumab	PD-1	Melanoma, NSCLC, MSI-H cancers, squamous cell head and neck, urothelial bladder cancer, Hodgkin's disease
• Daratumumab	CD38	Multiple myeloma

Abbreviations: Her2, human epidermal growth factor receptor 2; VEGF, vascular endothelial growth factor; GBM, glioblastoma multiformae; EGFR, epidermal growth factor receptor; CTLA-4, cytotoxic T lymphocyte associated protein 4; PD-1, programmed cell death protein-1; NSCLC, non-small-cell lung cancer; MSI-H, microsatellite instability-high.

Table 1.2 Examples of small molecule tyrosine kinase inhibitors (TKIs) in oncology

Small molecule TKIs	Targets	Malignancies where active
• Imatinib	Bcr-abl kinase	CML, GIST
• Erlotinib	EGFR kinase	NSCLC, pancreatic cancer
• Crizotinib	ALK	ALK positive NSCLC
• Sorafenib	Multi-targeted	HCC, renal cell
• Sunitinib	Multi-targeted	Renal cell, GIST, pNET
• Regorafenib	Multi-targeted	Colon, GIST, HCC

Abbreviations: Bcr-abl, Breakpoint cluster region on chromosome 22-Abelson on chromosome 9; EGFR, epidermal growth factor receptor; ALK, anaplastic lymphoma kinase; CML, chronic myelogenous leukemia; GIST, gastrointestinal stromal tumor; HCC, hepatocellular cancer; pNET, pancreatic neuroendocrine cancer.

Systemic Therapy in Oncology

In using systemic therapy, one of the first things the oncologist has to determine is whether the goal of treatment in a particular patient is cure or palliation. When cure is the goal, it raises the stakes and there is usually little room for deviation from the regimen, schedule, and dosing that have been derived from clinical trials. Any experimental agent used in this setting therefore is usually additive, that is, used in addition to rather than in place of the standard therapy. On the other hand, when cure is not possible there is generally greater flexibility with the treatment and this is typically the proving ground for new, experimental therapies that if found to be safe and effective not only help improve outcomes in this setting, but also become candidates for being moved up to be tested in curable subsets of patients.

Chemotherapy for Cure

Patients can potentially be cured and are treated with that intent when a solid tumor can be surgically removed with clear margins or an available chemotherapeutic regimen is curative by itself or in selected situations where chemotherapy used concurrently with radiation can eradicate all tumor cells. Let us look briefly at each of these scenarios in current practice.

- *As primary therapy*: Chemotherapy combinations can cure certain malignancies regardless of whether they are localized or not (**Table 1.3**). Additionally, there are small subsets of patients (typically 5% or less) with melanoma, renal cell cancer or small cell lung cancer that can be cured with systemic therapy.[20,21,22]

- *As adjuvant therapy*: Patients with solid tumors that are able to undergo complete surgical resection are considered potentially cured. However, it has been noted that many of these patients have disease recurrence particularly if they had locally advanced tumors with involvement of lymph nodes. Administration of systemic chemotherapy in such patients can eradicate micrometastases and thereby increase the chance of cure. This was first successfully proven in breast cancer and then colon cancer starting in the 1970s[23,24] and has now become the standard of care for these as well as several other cancers (**Table 1.4**).

- *As concomitant therapy with radiation*: When chemotherapy is used with radiation, it serves as a sensitizer to the cytotoxic effects of the latter such that the two together produce a greater tumor kill than either one by itself. Although this is true for most solid tumors, the response in squamous cell cancers treated in this way is sufficiently robust to be potentially curative without any further intervention such as surgery. (**Table 1.5**) This is particularly helpful in areas

Table 1.3 Malignancies that are curable with chemotherapy

- Acute lymphocytic leukemia
- Acute myeloid leukemia
- Hodgkin lymphoma
- Subsets of non-Hodgkin lymphoma
- Germ cell tumors (including testicular cancer)
- Ovarian cancer
- Choriocarcinoma

Table 1.4 Malignancies for which adjuvant chemotherapy after surgery ± radiation therapy increases cure rates

- Breast cancer
- Colorectal cancer
- Cervical cancer
- Gastric cancer
- Head and neck cancers
- Pancreatic cancer
- Melanoma
- Non–small cell lung cancer
- Ovarian cancer
- Osteosarcoma
- Anaplastic astrocytoma

Table 1.5 Malignancies that are potentially curable with concurrent chemotherapy and radiation

- Squamous cell cancers of the head and neck
- Squamous cell cancer of the esophagus
- Squamous cell cancer of the cervix
- Squamous cell cancer of the anal canal

such as the head and neck and the anal canal where avoiding surgery spares patients from serious cosmetic and functional consequences.[25,26]

Chemotherapy for Palliation

When cure is not achievable by available modalities described above, the goal of treatment is palliation, which involves controlling the disease to improve quality of life (QOL) and prolonging survival. This is usually the case in most solid tumors that are not amenable to surgery due to locally advanced or metastatic disease or both and for which primary chemotherapy is not curative. Since these patients are not cured with a limited course of treatment, they are typically on long-term systemic therapy to control their disease. This is much like the management paradigm for other chronic and incurable diseases such as hypertension or diabetes except that the agents used for treating oncologic disease are usually more toxic and do not work indefinitely. The survival of responding patients is improved with this approach although depending on tumor type and biology, it can vary substantially from a few months in most pancreatic or lung cancer patients, for example, to several years in some breast cancer patients. Given this, maintaining a good QOL takes on a greater significance in these patients as compared to those being treated for a limited time for cure. The goals of controlling the disease and optimizing QOL have to be carefully balanced since most of the available therapies, including many of the newer targeted ones, have the potential for causing significant toxicities. These can range from myelosuppression resulting in risk for infection or bleeding to a host of other multisystem toxicities such as fatigue, nausea, vomiting, diarrhea, oral mucositis, hand–foot syndrome, acneiform skin rashes, electrolyte disturbances, organ dysfunction (heart, liver, lungs, and other organs) as well as a variety of autoimmune complications of the newer immunotherapies. There are several strategies used by medical oncologists to achieve and maintain the balance between disease control and optimal QOL for as long as possible. These are summarized below.

- *Dose and schedule adjustments*: Besides using supportive and symptomatic measures as detailed in **Table 1.6**, modifying the dose and schedule of the chemotherapeutic agents is a key strategy in maintaining the balance between disease control and QOL. Often, the first intervention is to reduce the dose of the offending agent(s). Sometimes, the schedule can be modified to make the treatment more tolerable such as, for example, going from 2 weeks on and 1 week off to every other week administration.[27]
- *Induction with "aggressive" regimen, followed by maintenance with "gentler" regimen*: An example of this is the use of FOLFOX ± Bevacizumab for initial therapy in metastatic colorectal cancer and then stopping oxaliplatin after a maximal response is obtained or the patient develops significant peripheral neuropathy. The patient can then be maintained on 5FU and leucovorin ± Bevacizumab, which is likely to be better tolerated over a longer period of time.[28,29,30]
- *Use of adjunctive modalities (radioembolization, stereotactic radiation therapy) to maximize time on "gentler" maintenance systemic therapies*: This is particularly helpful in cases where a patient with widely metastatic disease who is doing well on low intensity maintenance therapy has evidence of disease progression in one or two isolated lesions with no change in the rest of the disease. This probably occurs as a result of new mutations in those metastatic sites and if these isolated areas can be embolized or ablated, the patient may be able to continue on the same regimen instead of having to change to an alternative with potentially more side effects and adverse impact on QOL.
- *Supportive/symptomatic measures*: These are not only useful in improving the QOL for patients being treated with palliative intent, but also very important in the safe delivery of the full intensity of therapy in patients being treated with curative intent (**Table 1.6**).
- *Drug holidays (usually brief, ~2–4 weeks)*: Most studies have suggested that brief drug holidays in patients with metastatic cancer with well-controlled disease do not adversely affect the overall therapeutic efficacy and survival.[31] Such breaks give many patients a much-needed respite from the side effects of treatment and can also be opportunities for them to enjoy quality time with family and friends during special events.

Table 1.6 Supportive care in oncology

- Prophylaxis and treatment of chemotherapy-induced nausea/vomiting (CINV): *Dexamethasone, 5-HT3 inhibitors (e.g., ondansetron), neurokinin-1 antagonist (aprepitant), other anti-emetics (e.g., promethazine, metoclopramide)*
- Prophylactic growth factor support to prevent neutropenia in highly myelosuppressive regimens: *Filgrastim or pegfilgrastim*
- Prophylaxis and treatment of cancer-related thrombosis: *Typically with low molecular weight heparin rather than warfarin or rivaroxaban*
- Symptomatic treatment of unique side effects of chemotherapy agents: *Antidiarrheal agents (for irinotecan), Neurontin and analgesics (for neuropathy related to taxanes, platinums and vinca alkaloids)*
- Pain management: *Analgesics per WHO (World Health Organization) ladder (although narcotic analgesics are used quite commonly in treating pain in cancer patients)*
- Psychological support and intervention as needed: *Counseling, anxiolytics, antidepressants*

Summary

The use of systemic therapy has evolved over the last half century to become an important component of the treatment of cancer that has helped improve survival and even achieve cure in patients with a variety of malignancies. This is often done in conjunction with other anti-cancer modalities such as surgery and radiation therapy to achieve the best outcomes. Over the last couple of decades, interventional radiology has become an increasingly important modality in this context, not only with regard to providing diagnostic tissue samples and optimal vascular access but also for highly selective and targeted delivery of cytotoxic agents, including, more recently, oncolytic viruses.

References

1. Marshall EK Jr. Historical perspectives in chemotherapy. In: Golding A, Hawking IF, eds. Advances in Chemotherapy. Vol 1. New York, NY: Academic Press; 1964:1–8

2. Li MC, Hertz R, Bergenstal DM. Therapy of choriocarcinoma and related trophoblastic tumors with folic acid and purine antagonists. N Engl J Med 1958;259(2):66–74

3. Freireich EJ, Karon M, Frei E III. Quadruple combination therapy (VAMP) for acute lymphocytic leukemia of childhood. Proc Am Assoc Cancer Res 1964;5:20

4. Holland JF. Hopes for tomorrow versus realities of today: therapy and prognosis in acute lymphocytic leukemia of childhood. Pediatrics 1970;45(2):191–193

5. Li MC, Whitmore WF, Goldbey RB, Grabstald H. Effects of combined drug therapy on metastatic cancer of the testis. JAMA 1960;174:1291–1299

6. Einhorn LH, Donohue J. Cis-diamminedichloroplatinum, vinblastine, and bleomycin combination chemotherapy in disseminated testicular cancer. Ann Intern Med 1977;87(3):293–298

7. DeVita VT Jr, Serpick AA, Carbone PP. Combination chemotherapy in the treatment of advanced Hodgkin's disease. Ann Intern Med 1970;73(6):881–895

8. DeVita VT Jr, Canellos GP, Chabner B, Schein P, Hubbard SP, Young RC. Advanced diffuse histiocytic lymphoma, a potentially curable disease. Lancet 1975;1(7901):248–250

9. DeVita VT, Schein PS. The use of drugs in combination for the treatment of cancer: rationale and results. N Engl J Med 1973;288(19):998–1006

10. McLaughlin P, Grillo-López AJ, Link BK, et al. Rituximab chimeric anti-CD20 monoclonal antibody therapy for relapsed indolent lymphoma: half of patients respond to a four-dose treatment program. J Clin Oncol 1998;16(8):2825–2833

11. Sousou T, Friedberg J. Rituximab in indolent lymphomas. Semin Hematol 2010;47(2):133–142

12. Eiermann W; International Herceptin Study Group. Trastuzumab combined with chemotherapy for the treatment of HER2-positive metastatic breast cancer: pivotal trial data. Ann Oncol 2001;12:S57–S62

13. Bartsch R, Wenzel C, Steger GG. Trastuzumab in the management of early and advanced stage breast cancer. Biologics 2007;1(1):19–31

14. Druker BJ, Sawyers CL, Kantarjian H, et al. Activity of a specific inhibitor of the BCR-ABL tyrosine kinase in the blast crisis of chronic myeloid leukemia and acute lymphoblastic leukemia with the Philadelphia chromosome. N Engl J Med 2001;344(14):1038–1042

15. Krause DS, Van Etten RA. Tyrosine kinases as targets for cancer therapy. N Engl J Med 2005;353(2):172–187

16. Mansi L, Pages F, Adotevi O. Immune checkpoint inhibitors. Rev Cell Bio Mol Medicine 2016;2:70–99

17. Postow MA, Callahan MK, Wolchok JD. Immune checkpoint blockade in cancer therapy. J Clin Oncol 2015;33(17):1974–1982

18. Johnson DB, Puzanov I, Kelley MC. Talimogene laherparepvec (T-VEC) for the treatment of advanced melanoma. Immunotherapy 2015;7(6):611–619

19. Gill S, June CH. Going viral: chimeric antigen receptor T-cell therapy for hematological malignancies. Immunol Rev 2015;263(1):68–89

20. Atkins MB, Lotze MT, Dutcher JP, et al. High-dose recombinant interleukin 2 therapy for patients with metastatic melanoma: analysis of 270 patients treated between 1985 and 1993. J Clin Oncol 1999;17(7):2105–2116

21. Dillman RO, Barth NM, VanderMolen LA, Mahdavi K, McClure SE. Should high-dose interleukin-2 still be the preferred treatment for patients with metastatic melanoma? Cancer Biother Radiopharm 2012;27(6):337–343

22. Shablak A, Sikand K, Shanks JH, Thistlethwaite F, Spencer-Shaw A, Hawkins RE. High-dose interleukin-2 can produce a high rate of response and durable remissions in appropriately selected patients with metastatic renal cancer. J Immunother 2011;34(1):107–112

23. Fisher B, Carbone P, Economou SG, et al. 1-Phenylalanine mustard (L-PAM) in the management of primary breast cancer. A report of early findings. N Engl J Med 1975;292(3):117–122

24. Wolmark N, Rockette H, Fisher B, et al. The benefit of leucovorin-modulated fluorouracil as postoperative adjuvant therapy for primary colon cancer: re-sults from National Surgical Adjuvant Breast and Bowel Project protocol C-03. J Clin Oncol 1993;11(10):1879–1887

25. Nigro ND, Vaitkevicius VK, Considine B Jr. Combined therapy for cancer of the anal canal: a preliminary report. Dis Colon Rectum 1974;17(3):354–356

26. Wolf GT, Fisher SG, Hong WK, et al. Department of Veterans Affairs Laryngeal Cancer Study Group. Induction chemotherapy plus radiation compared with surgery plus radiation in patients with advanced laryngeal cancer. N Engl J Med 1991;324(24):1685–1690

27. Krishna K, Blazer MA, Wei L, et al. Modified gemcitabine and nab-paclitaxel in patients with metastatic pancreatic cancer (MPC): a single-institution expe-rience. ASCO Gastrointestinal Cancers Symposium. January 15–17, 2015; San Francisco, CA

28. Tournigand C, Cervantes A, Figer A, et al. OPTIMOX1: a randomized study of FOLFOX4 or FOLFOX7 with oxaliplatin in a stop-and-Go fashion in advanced colorectal cancer—a GERCOR study. J Clin Oncol 2006;24(3):394–400

29. Chibaudel B, Maindrault-Goebel F, Lledo G, et al. Can chemotherapy be discontinued in unresectable metastatic colorectal cancer? The GERCOR OPTIMOX2 Study. J Clin Oncol 2009;27(34):5727–5733

30. Hochster HS. Stop and go: yes or no? J Clin Oncol 2009;27(34):5677–5679

31. Labianca R, Sobrero A, Isa L, et al; Italian Group for the Study of Gastroin-testinal Cancer-GISCAD. Intermittent versus continuous chemotherapy in advanced colorectal cancer: a randomised 'GISCAD' trial. Ann Oncol 2011;22(5):1236–1242

2 Essentials of Surgical Oncology

Robert C. G. Martin II

Introduction

Surgery is an essential part of the treatment for patients with many types of cancer.[1–4] Achieving the best results, however, often requires the coordinated efforts of an interdisciplinary team (multidisciplinary concept). Surgical oncologists are uniquely trained not only in the techniques of cancer surgery, but also in how surgery fits in to the big picture of cancer care.[5] Rather than viewing surgical procedures in isolation, surgical oncologists consider operations within the context of treatment plans that may incorporate chemotherapy, radiation therapy, and/or alternative approaches before, during, and after surgery. A surgical oncologist establishes a strong collaborative disease management program with other cancer-related disciplines to offer patients with a wide array of cancer treatments at the right time for the best chance for long-term quality of life.

Education is an essential part of surgical oncology that commonly involves interdisciplinary cancer conferences on breast, liver, pancreatic, biliary, and gastrointestinal (GI) malignancies, which are usually held on a weekly basis. These conferences serve an important role in optimizing patients' multidisciplinary care as well as educating students, residents, and fellows about approaches to cancer care. Even more importantly, from the patients' perspective, these conferences are the forum for cancer teams to plan the management of complex cases, review the results from surgery, determine the need for additional postoperative treatment, and consider patients for whom effective standard therapy is not available for entry into clinical trials.[6]

Surgery, while the best treatment available, does not yet offer a sure cure for many cancer patients; an active program of clinical and translational research, bringing the newest promising developments from laboratories, is integral to any surgical oncology program. Studies in early cancer detection, tumor markers, cancer genetics, environmental risk factors, minimally invasive surgical techniques, nonsurgical tumor ablation, downstaging of advanced cancer to allow for surgical resection, transplantation for tumors, anesthesia for cancer surgery, adjuvant treatment to prevent cancer recurrence, tumor vaccines, gene therapy, and nonchemotherapy treatment of advanced cancer are all components in surgical oncology.

Historical Perspective

For the first half of the 20th century, cancer was essentially a surgical disease. By the mid-20th century, with the development of radiation therapy subsequent to discovery of X-rays and chemotherapy, the treatment of cancer changed dramatically. The significant expansion of medical oncology and radiation oncology has made evident that cancer is not a surgical-only disease, but one best treated with a multimodality therapy. The concept of surgical oncology first arose in the 1960s to better differentiate between medical oncologists and surgeons who did not specialize in oncology.

The essential principles of surgical therapy are established on several key factors.

- Identifying and diagnosing of suspicious masses.
- Staging of established cancers.
- Providing curative resection of primary and several metastatic cancers.
- Prevention of surgery by risk-reducing surgery.
- Evaluating the concept of debulking malignancies as part of a multimodality therapy.
- Providing surgical palliation of incurable patients.

The role of surgery in the treatment of cancer was initiated with John Hunter (1728–1793), the father of scientific surgery.[7] He first described the concept that cancer could be a localized process and amenable to surgical therapy with the discussion of the removal of regional lymph node disease. As surgery became safer and more feasible and as extensive understanding of anatomy and pathology finalized with the introduction of general anesthesia in 1842, surgery became the cornerstone of cancer treatment. It allowed the field to move beyond the superficial tumors and foray into intra-abdominal malignancies. The initial description of major intra-abdominal procedures began in the next few decades with the description of partial gastrectomy (Bill Roth in 1881), colectomy (Weir in 1885), radical mastectomy (Halstead in 1891), and abdominal perineal resection (Myles in 1908). For the next several decades, surgery was the mainstay of cancer therapy with the mortality and morbidity of surgery limited by the potential of long-term palliation and disease-free survival. This was accompanied by significant growth in cytotoxic systemic chemotherapy[8] as well as radiation oncology,[9] and with this the field of oncology began to transform rapidly.

With these developments, the role of the surgical oncologist evolved as well and it continues to do so in the management of cancer as we gain additional knowledge in tumor immunology, genetics, and molecular biology (tumor immunology). Whereas historically and even up to 10 years ago surgery was almost always the first step in therapy, now with the escalating use of neoadjuvant therapies, both systemic and localized, surgical therapy or consolidative surgery is now the second- or third-line treatment after the biology of the disease and the physiology of the patient have been established. This has required surgeons to become extensively knowledgeable in systemic chemotherapy, local regional therapies, as well as radiation oncology.

Modern Surgical Oncology

Today, the surgical oncologist is often called upon not only to diagnose, stage, and treat cancer, but also to coordinate the care of the patient among the multiple disciplines within oncology. The treatment of cancer is constantly changing as new technologies and therapies emerge. Thus, a surgical oncologist and the training of surgical oncologists place a significant emphasis on ensuring that board-certified surgical oncologists have a very strong understanding of chemotherapy, radiation therapy, cancer biology, genetics, immunology, and epidemiology. Because the study of surgical oncology covers such a wide array of topics, specifically by organ sites, it is not uncommon for certain surgical oncologists to further subspecialize into a specific organ or range of organs around their focus.

Surgical anatomy is critical to any surgical oncologist or hepatobiliary surgeon who takes keen interest in hepatic malignancies and they must have acute understanding of the surgical anatomy of the liver. It is well established that there is *no* normal anatomy when it comes to surgical anatomy of the GI tract, liver, or pancreas due predominantly to the significant anatomic variations that occur, the distortion that tumors can induce from angiogenesis as well as from direct compression, and because of the significant effects that other prior systemic chemotherapy, percutaneous interventions, or hepatic arterial interventions can induce. It is essential to have a clear understanding of the anatomy based on the more common vascular outflow and vascular inflow and biliary outflow in addition to the hepatic outflow. However, the key is understanding that "normal" anatomy is present at best only in 60% of patients, with a large majority having a variant anatomy; therefore, understanding and identifying the variant anatomy during preoperative imaging is important prior to any type of surgical intervention.

The main focus of surgical oncology should be understanding that surgical therapy is the treatment of choice for long-term disease-free control of solid neoplasms. Surgery has its recognized limits in regard to its application and ability of patients to tolerate that type of treatment modality, and it is predominantly focused on understanding the biology of that malignant solid neoplasm. In a majority of all upper GI and hepatopancreatobiliary malignancies, a true multimodality therapy has become the standard of care. The role of the surgical oncologist continues to be focused on being a consultant and collaborator in the multidisciplinary management of patients, organizer, and leader commonly of prospective multidisciplinary tumor boards, cancer programs and committees, as well as continued emphasis on prospective clinical trials.

Prevention, Diagnosis, and Staging

Additional focus within surgical oncology is clearly around prevention and early detection since it is well established that earlier-stage malignancies will require less invasive and less extensive surgical therapy. There are certain subsets of GI malignancies (familial adenomatous polyposis [FAP], hereditary nonpolyposis colorectal cancer [HNPCC], breast cancer [BRCA], and others) in which risk-reducing surgical resection has been found to reduce the overall incidence of that malignancy as well as significantly impact long-term overall survival of these patients. When considering a high-risk surgery, it is critical to make an extensive evaluation of the true lifetime risk of the patient, quality-of-life effects from the surgery, and the emotional effects that may occur.

Additional roles of surgical oncology include cancer diagnosis and staging through high-quality imaging as well as tissue acquisition. There are several solid organs in which tissue diagnosis is both challenging and met with a high degree of false-negative results, especially in regard to hepatopancreatobiliary disease. There are times when definitive high-quality cross-sectional imaging provides a greater degree of accuracy in diagnosing and establishing optimal treatment algorithms than in tissue acquisition. Common examples of this include hepatocellular carcinoma, pancreatic adenocarcinoma, and metastatic neuroendocrine disease. At times, there can be an overemphasis on obtaining needle or tissue diagnosis with simple higher-quality thin-cut triphasic computed tomography (CT) scan; however, dynamic imaging should be utilized and should be implemented if a patient has had a standard scan recently. It is not uncommon that high-quality thin-cut triphasic CT scans will change the stage of the patient, by upstaging nearly 40% of all upper GI and hepatopancreatobiliary malignancies. Surgical oncologists can provide quality assurance and ensure that appropriate and high-quality triphasic or dynamic imaging is utilized prior to initiating any type of palliative or therapeutic modality. It is essential for both optimal prognosis and optimal timing of therapy that the highest quality of staging is implemented in patients prior to therapy regardless of whether poor-quality imaging has been obtained recently. It is not uncommon for surgical oncologists to work extensively with insurance companies through a peer-to-peer review, educating them about the need of high-quality imaging regardless of the timing of the last scans because of high incidence of upstaging of patients with certain types of solid malignancies.

It is this high-quality staging in combination with a patient's underlying comorbidities and functional performance status that will allow a surgical oncologist to decide on the timing of surgical resectability as well as optimal timing of neoadjuvant or induction-based therapy. It has become far more of an accurate predictor of underlying outcomes to utilize functional physiologic status and frailty scores far more than simple age given the wide range of functional status that patients from age 50 to 85 years can have with GI and hepatopancreatobiliary malignancies. Age alone has been found to be both inaccurate and insensitive in predicting a patient's underlying physiologic reserve and the ability to tolerate any type of modality of therapy regardless of the access of delivery. The desires of the patient's family are essential to outline not just the initial treatment but also, more importantly, the whole range and algorithm of treatment that commonly can last between 6 and 9 months for upper GI and hepatopancreatobiliary malignancies.

Multimodality Therapy

This ability to evaluate the patient is one of the major challenges of the surgical oncologist in that accurate identification of patients who can be treated effectively with appropriate multimodality therapy that is safe and effective and, most importantly, allows the patient to regain or maintain their underlying quality of life during therapy is at times hard. This takes constant communication among the multidisciplinary team and other oncologic specialties as well as constant evaluation at 2- to 3-month intervals to ensure that optimal therapeutic delivery and optimal responses are achieved. It is this initial therapy that allows the second major challenge of the surgical oncologist to be evaluated, which is the timing of consolidative therapy. Consolidative local therapy that is either surgical resection, radiation therapy, or local ablative therapy provides similar goals through different methods of action with the underlying treatment success being definitive local control of a primary tumor. There are widespread risks and benefits as to which of the above-mentioned procedures are optimal based on the disease process and disease location, which are outside the scope of this chapter. However, it is imperative that the surgical oncologist and all other treating multidisciplinary physicians are in agreement as to when that consolidative therapy should be performed and what the true benefits are. One of the single greatest challenges for current multidisciplinary teams that are practicing in this century is that there are a lot of "can therapies" that can be delivered to patients, but it is far more imperative that the multidisciplinary team truly thinks this therapy should be delivered. Continuing to practice a "can" therapeutic decision making will lead to significant failures defined as unacceptable short disease-free intervals, unacceptable higher percentages of recurrences, and, probably, most importantly, reduction in overall survival.

The third major challenge for the surgical oncologist is defining the use, timing, and duration of adjuvant therapy after this consolidative therapy has been delivered. Understanding the types of approved adjuvant therapies and most importantly understanding the risk potential of these patients as to who truly is at high risk for recurrence and, more importantly, who can benefit from this adjuvant therapy is imperative for the surgical oncologist to understand, guide, and educate their patients in collaboration with other multidisciplinary physicians.

References

1. North DA, Groeschl RT, Sindram D, et al. Microwave ablation for hepatic malignancies: a call for standard reporting and outcomes. Am J Surg 2014;208(2):284–294

2. Martin RC II, Loehle J, Scoggins CR, McMasters KM. Kentucky hepatoma: epidemiologic variant or same problem in a different region? Arch Surg 2007;142(5):431–436, discussion 436–437

3. Bower M, Metzger T, Robbins K, et al. Surgical downstaging and neo-adjuvant therapy in metastatic colorectal carcinoma with irinotecan drug-eluting beads: a multi-institutional study. HPB (Oxford) 2010;12(1):31–36

4. Whitney R, Tatum C, Hahl M, et al. Safety of hepatic resection in metastatic disease to the liver after yttrium-90 therapy. J Surg Res 2011;166(2):236–240

5. Are C, Berman RS, Wyld L, Cummings C, Lecoq C, Audisio RA. Global curriculum in surgical oncology. Ann Surg Oncol 2016;23(6):1782–1795

6. Martin RC II, Polk HC Jr, Jaques DP. Does additional surgical training increase participation in randomized controlled trials? Am J Surg 2003;185(3):239–243

7. Toledo-Pereyra LH. Birth of scientific surgery. John Hunter versus Joseph Lister as the father or founder of scientific surgery. J Invest Surg 2010;23(1):6–11

8. Gustavsson B, Carlsson G, Machover D, et al. A review of the evolution of systemic chemotherapy in the management of colorectal cancer. Clin Colorectal Cancer 2015;14(1):1–10

9. Connell PP, Hellman S. Advances in radiotherapy and implications for the next century: a historical perspective. Cancer Res 2009;69(2):383–392

3 Essentials of Radiation Oncology

Andrew S. Kennedy

Introduction to Radiation Oncology

Radiation oncology is the medical use of ionizing radiation in cancer treatment to control malignant cells. Ionizing radiation damages the DNA (deoxyribonucleic acid) of cells, either directly or indirectly, by forming free radicals and reactive oxygen species. Whereas healthy normal cells are differentiated and can repair themselves, in cancer cells DNA damage is inherited through cell division and the accumulation of this damage to malignant cells results in cell death. Ionizing radiation can be produced by electron, photon, proton, neutron, or ion beams. Provided below is a short summary of the establishment of radiation oncology, the overall structure of its governing bodies, a definition of the scope of practice of radiation oncology, and the primary treatment approaches that are employed.

Brief History of the Specialty

The field of radiation therapy (RT; also known as radiotherapy and radiation oncology) arose shortly after Wilhelm Rontgen discovered X-rays in 1895. The use of X-rays was rapidly taken up by physicians for such purposes as diagnosing broken bones and locating foreign objects in patients. However, in 1896, Antoine-Henri Becquerel recognized that certain elements spontaneously emitted rays or subatomic particles from matter; this property came to be known as radioactivity. In their experiments, which led to the identification of polonium and radium, Pierre and Marie Curie observed radium destroying diseased cells. This was the first indication that radiation was a boon not only to disease diagnosis, but also to treatment.

In the early 1900s, the field of RT expanded quickly, spawning a new era in medical treatment and research. Physicians initially tested exposure to X-rays and based their clinical practice on their observations. Although the mechanism of action for radiation effects had not yet been identified, reports of tumor control or regression began to fund the scientific literature. Researchers were optimistic about the benefits of radiation, but wary of its possible harms.

Roentgenology, as it was then known, assumed a role in World War I, wherein radiologic equipment was used in field hospitals, and French and American soldiers were trained to take X-rays; thus, the demand for radiologic service and technology continued to rise. In time, many physicians purchased X-ray machines for their office practices, and several even announced their specialty as radiology. Between the world wars, physicists and biologists continued to discover the mechanisms of radiation and how to measure the dosages accurately. Higher energy X-ray machines and new radium devices came on the market.

Skip to the 1960s, when megavoltage treatment machines, known as linear accelerators or Linacs, were introduced. Linacs could produce uniform doses of high-energy beams, allowing the penetration treatment of tumors deep inside the body, yet sparing excessive damage to overlying skin and other normal tissues. In the 1970s and 1980s, computers could be used to plan treatment. The advent of new imaging technologies, including magnetic resonance imaging (MRI) and position emission tomography (PET), moved RT from 3D conformal to intensity-modulated radiation therapy (IMRT) and image-guided radiation therapy (IGRT). IMRT with different intensities of radiation beams allows the simultaneous delivery of different doses of radiation. Higher doses of radiation can be delivered to tumors and lower doses to nearby healthy tissue. A distinct benefit of IGRT is in allowing the radiation oncologist to image the tumor immediately before and during the treatment, allowing clinicians to better see and target tumors. This has resulted in better treatment outcomes, more organ preservation, and fewer side effects.

Governing Bodies of Radiation Oncology

In the United States, the field of radiation oncology is governed by two primary groups: the American College of Radiology (ACR) and the American Society for Therapeutic Radiology and Oncology (ASTRO). ACR, with more than 30,000 members, is the principal organization of radiologists, radiation oncologists, and clinical medical physicists. The college is a nonprofit professional society whose primary purposes are to advance the science of radiology, improve radiologic services to the patient, study the socioeconomic aspects of the practice of radiology, and encourage continuing education for radiologists, radiation oncologists, medical physicists, and persons practicing in allied professional fields.

ASTRO became its own entity, endeavoring to, among other efforts, assist with continuing medical educational opportunities and standards for educating RT trainees. In the 1990s, the society began to communicate the specialty's goals and achievements to the general public, compose strategic 5-year plans to achieve its goals, represent member interests in legislative and regulatory spheres, and foster leadership growth within its ranks. In 1998, ASTRO became its own independently managed society with its own headquarters in Fairfax, VA. ASTRO then increased involvement in socioeconomic issues and expanded efforts in outcomes research. In the new millennium, ASTRO has ingrown its efforts in health policy and government relations, as well as Medicare and Medicaid issues. ASTRO continues to focus on issues of importance to its members, such as technology advances, treatment regimens, communications dissemination initiatives, and newer issues such as the importance of radiobiology. ASTRO also continues to work with other medical organizations and specialties to share research and information. In 2008, the society changed its name to the American Society for Radiation Oncology, still retaining the acronym ASTRO.

ACR periodically defines new practice parameters and technical standards for radiologic practice to help advance the science of radiology and to improve the quality of service. ACR and ASTRO collaborate on scope of practice and practice parameters.

Definition of Radiation Oncology Scope of Practice

Radiation oncology is one of the primary disciplines, along with surgical and medical oncology, involved in cancer treatment. RT is a cornerstone of cancer care and is one of the most powerful therapies in oncologic practice, with the capability of preserving organ and function while providing the potential for cure. RT is the use of ionizing radiation to destroy or inhibit the growth of malignant tissues. It is also used in selected clinical situations to inhibit the growth or modulate the function of tissues in certain benign diseases. Separate practice parameters and standards define the appropriate use of external beam therapy, brachytherapy, and other therapies using radionuclides. RT with either curative or palliative intent is used to treat up to 60% of all patients with cancer.[1]

In the current economic environment, the widespread use of new and more expensive technologies has reduced the cost of RT relative to that of systemic therapies. Finding and then justifying its appropriate use using the tools of comparative effectiveness have become a major and urgent responsibility for investigators.[2]

Early in 2011 ASTRO's Board of Directors began formally discussing the future of the basic sciences of radiation oncology. Its focus was the current state and potential future direction of basic research within the specialty. In August 2011, a Cancer Biology/Radiation Biology Task Force (TF) was initiated and charged with developing an accurate snapshot of the current state of basic (preclinical) research in radiation oncology, its relevance to modern radiation oncology clinical practice, and the education of trainees and attending physicians in the biological sciences. The TF was further charged with making suggestions as to critical areas of biological basic research investigation that might be most likely to maintain and build further the scientific foundation and vitality of radiation oncology as an independent and vibrant medical specialty.[3]

Main Radiation Oncology Treatment Approaches

Radiation used in the treatment of malignant cells can be directed into the body from either an internal or external source. In the past two decades, technologic advancements in radiation oncology and diagnostic radiology have allowed for innovative approaches to therapy. The two main available approaches are external beam radiation therapy (EBRT) and brachytherapy. A radiation oncologist may have at his/her disposal external beam treatment equipment that provides beams other than conventional photon and electron beams (e.g., proton beams). Special expertise on the part of the radiation oncologist as well as the physics and therapy staff is required for safely using this treatment equipment. Brachytherapy (radioembolization [RE]) may be used for many sites and may be delivered with either low-dose-rate or high-dose-rate techniques.

Powerful technology growth in the modern era, such as computer hardware upgrades, including megavoltage linear accelerators, and software programs that enable conversion of computed tomography (CT) or MRI datasets into three-dimensional (3D) virtual patients have meant expanding effects in radiation oncology therapies. With accurate 3D models of the patient to work from and estimates in real time of radiation dose deposition within the patient, radiation oncologists can attempt to deliver the higher doses of radiation that have a chance to control tumors while sparing the nonmalignant cells. Technologic advances in EBRT and brachytherapy as well as the commercial availability of radioactive microsphere products allow a broader spectrum of treatment to those with primary and metastatic disease (**Fig. 3.1**; **Fig. 3.2**).

Continuous low-dose radiotherapy is the type of brachytherapy delivered by yttrium-90 (90Y) microspheres. Compared with external beam (via modern linear accelerators), which is high dose (500 cGy/min), pulsatile (once/24 h), and delivered 5 d/wk, RE delivers effective dose rate radiation at low dose (50 cGy/min), continuously (every second), and 7 d/wk for 14 days.

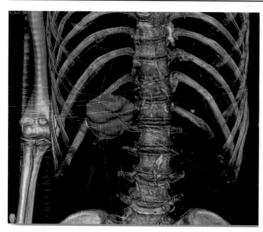

Fig. 3.1 Digital reconstructed radiograph from a computed tomography scan. A metastatic colon cancer deposit is seen in the right hepatic lobe (blue object). The liver itself and other soft tissues are transparent to facilitate visualization of the tumor and planned stereotactic body radiotherapy beams (blue lines).

Physics of Radiation Oncology

The seminal event in the tumor cell targeted by radiation is ionization of the DNA located in the nucleus. Although many potential targets in the malignant cell can produce radiation damage, the cessation of reproductive capacity is the true goal of RT. The direct effect on DNA—the photon or β particle striking one of the two DNA strands—causes irreversible damage and occurs in just 25% of lethal interactions. The indirect radiation effect on DNA, which leads to cell death in 75% of encounters, involves a water molecule–absorbing radiation energy, ejection of a Compton electron from the outer shell of the oxygen atom, and the creation of a free radical. The highly unstable and reactive free radical develops within 4 nm of the DNA strand, which leads to either a single-strand or a double-strand DNA break. If unrepaired, the cell will lose reproductive integrity, and die either via apoptosis or after a few additional cell divisions. The presence of oxygen is critical for the successful creation of free radical damage near to the DNA.[4]

Radiation that is of sufficient energy to cause ionization of cellular contents is used therapeutically and is either an electromagnetic or a particulate energy form. Electromagnetic energy, or photons, can be produced naturally by decay of radioactive isotopes (γ-rays) or by an electrical device accelerating electrons, which abruptly stop in a target, releasing energy (X-rays). Particulate energy most commonly used for cancer therapy is electrons (charge: –1; energy: 0.511 MeV [million electron volts]; mass: 9.109382910^{-31} kg), but others in limited use include protons (charge: +1; energy: 938.27231 MeV; mass: 1.67262310^{-27} kg, which is ~2,000 × electron), a-particles (helium ions), and neutrons (same mass as proton, no charge).

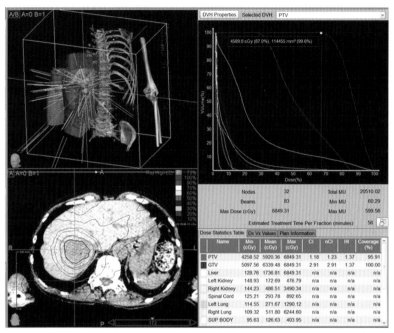

Fig. 3.2 Screenshot of the stereotactic body radiotherapy treatment planning software showing the final plan and radiation dose deposition in the body. The upper left panel is a three-dimensional reconstruction with cut-away view of liver and tumor, targeted by 83 beams of photons (blue lines). The upper right panel is a dose-volume histogram graph showing the amount of each organ receiving a percentage of the total radiation delivered to the tumor. It is also summarized in the lower right panel in table form. The lower left panel is an axial view with the radiation dose displayed as different-colored lines (isodose lines) around the targeted tumor. This tumor was given a total of 5,000 cGy from five individual fractions of 6-MV photons, one fraction of 1,000 cGy per day, in 5 consecutive days. Total treatment time each day was 56 minutes. A RECIST (Response Evaluation Criteria in Solid Tumors) 1.1 partial response was achieved.

External Beam Radiation Therapy

External beam RT delivers radiation outside the body; EBRT that employs X-rays is the most commonly used method for treating nearly all cancers. Photons, which are discrete packets of electromagnetic energy, cause cell damage or cell death via apoptosis, colliding with a cell and transferring a portion of energy to the cell. This interaction exchanges some energy to the cell, and the photon itself is deflected with a reduction in its energy. The energy absorbed by the cell will possibly create damage to the DNA, leading to cell death.

In the 1960s through early 1980s, external beam radiation was, in fact, the delivery of photons from radioactive decay of ^{60}Co. Although it yielded photon energies with sufficient penetrating power for most tumors, it could not be used for deep abdominal or pelvic tumors without delivering a much higher dose more superficially in normal tissues. In addition, the physical radiation beam itself possessed a relatively wide beam edge or penumbra, which made precise targeting impossible even at shallow depths of tissue.

Over the past 20 years, linear accelerators have replaced ^{60}Co machines virtually everywhere, generating photons by accelerating electrons approximately at the speed of light prior to striking a target. This activity converts kinetic energy and mass into electromagnetic energy photons. Linear accelerators generate photons of much higher energy than ^{60}Co and thus are able to reach any deep tumor in the body of most patients, without creating excessive hot spots or resulting in doses higher than that of the tumor along the photon path in the body. In absolute numbers, ^{60}Cot can deliver γ-rays (photons) of two energies, 1.17 MeV and 1.33 MeV; although some accelerators are capable of maximum photon energies of between 4 and 25 MeV, most centers use 6 to 18 MeV. Linear accelerators also can produce electron beams, which differ from photon beams in that electrons are particles with mass and charge, and thus have a finite range of tissue penetrance, allowing for treatment of more superficial tumors, while significantly sparing deeper normal tissues.

Brachytherapy

Not long after Roentgen discovered X-rays, *The Lancet* reported their medical use in January 1896.[4] Shortly after the turn of the century, Alexander Graham Bell suggested that radioactive isotopes be applied directly to tissues, and thus brachytherapy was born; the term originated from the Greek brachy, meaning "short range." Brachytherapy delivers sealed radioactive sources specifically in the target area of treatment. Dosage, determined during treatment planning, will depend on the site of the disease and if other modalities of treatment are being used in conjunction with RT.

Radioactive isotopes such as iridium (^{192}Ir), cesium (^{137}Cs), and iodine (^{125}I and ^{131}I) have been used extensively since the early 1900s as primary therapy and in addition to external beam radiation as a boost to the tumor. Brachytherapy attempts to spare normal regional tissues by delivering a high dose locally in the tumor, and although γ-radiation photons are primarily used, relatively low dose results at a distance from the tumor of several centimeters. The dose rate of radiation delivery via a brachytherapy isotope (50 cGy/h) is much lower than photons delivered by an accelerator (400–800 cGy/min).

Radioactive decay from an isotope that produces electrons (charge: –1) is termed β-decay. These particles are used in such products as radiolabeled antibodies used in hematologic malignancies or in higher energies, for bone metastases and thyroid malignancies. Currently, there is significant clinical use of pure β-emitting isotopes (no γ-photons emitted) yttrium (^{90}Y) and strontium (^{90}Sr) in brachytherapy in liver lesions and in coronary artery brachytherapy. An advantage and potential disadvantage of β-sources is that most of the effective radiation is delivered within 2 to 4 mm of the source, with virtually no radiation dose effect less than 1 cm away from the source. Because there are no γ-rays, nuclear medicine detectors cannot readily image pure sources, making localization of implanted sources problematic. Brachytherapy sources can be implanted via blood infusion or needle applicator, applied directly and sutured into place as a permanent implant, or placed temporarily (minutes to hours) within a catheter that is removed from the body.

Radiobiology

Radiobiology is a field of clinical and basic medical sciences that involves the study of the action of ionizing radiation on living things. In general, ionizing radiation is injurious and potentially lethal to living things; however, RT for the treatment of cancer may result in health benefits. On the other hand, RT may, in fact, induce cancer with a latent period of years or decades after exposure. High-dose RT can lead to radiation burns and/or rapid fatality through acute radiation syndrome. Other effects include radiation-induced lung injury, cataracts, and infertility.[5]

Some effects of ionizing radiation on human health are stochastic, meaning that their probability of occurrence increases with dose, while the severity is independent of dose.[5] Radiation-induced cancer, teratogenesis, cognitive decline, and heart disease are all examples of stochastic effects. Other conditions such as radiation burns, acute radiation syndrome, chronic radiation syndrome, and radiation-induced thyroiditis are deterministic, meaning they reliably occur above a threshold dose, and their severity increases with dose.[5] Deterministic effects are not necessarily more or less serious than stochastic effects; either can ultimately lead to a temporary nuisance or a fatality.

The spectrum of information related to diagnosis and management of radiation injuries and illnesses is vast. Exposures to ionizing radiation and internal contamination with radioactive materials can cause significant tissue damage and pathologic conditions. Therefore, medical imaging and radiotherapy employs tightly controlled doses.

An understanding of radiation effects in living tissues began at the turn of this century with observations of skin reaction, primarily erythema and breakdown[4] Since then, clinical experience has reported observations regarding normal and malignant tissue response and repair to ionizing radiation. The target of efficient cell killing is the DNA, with most cell death by irradiation resulting from unrepaired or misrepaired genomic injury and loss of reproductive ability. It has been estimated that in the presence of sufficient oxygen tension (>10 mm Hg),[4,6] any form of radiation (X-rays, γ-rays, charged or uncharged particles) will be absorbed and potentially interact directly or indirectly with the DNA. Approximately 75% of the damage to the DNA is indirect, with a photon striking a water molecule (water composes 80% of the cell). Kinetic energy from the incident photon is transferred to an orbital electron of the water molecule, ejecting it; the electron is then renamed a secondary electron. It can interact with a water molecule forming a free radical, which is highly reactive and breaks bonds in one of the DNA strands nearby. There also can be interaction of the secondary electron directly on the DNA strand, causing damage referred to as direct action.[4]

External Beam Radiation Therapy

Many clinical studies have correlated the radiobiology of treatment-absorbed doses and toxicity to organs at risk with tumor response. Dosimetry methods have evolved from the macroscopic approach at the organ level to voxel analysis, providing absorbed dose spatial distributions and dose-volume histograms (DVH). The effects of EBRT—such as volume effect, underlying disease influence, cumulative damage in parallel organs, and different tolerability of re-treatment—have also been observed in RE. Thus, EBRT and RE can be usefully compared. The radiobiologic models of normal tissue complication probability (NTCP) and tumor control probability, and/or the style (DVH concepts) used in EBRT have been introduced in RE.[7]

Brachytherapy

In the past two decades, RE with ^{90}Y microspheres has emerged as a safe and efficacious treatment modality for tumors in multiple settings, but particularly with unresectable primary and secondary liver malignancies. The rationale for using ^{90}Y is that both primary and secondary tumors in the liver receive their blood supply from the hepatic artery; the nontumoral liver is practically excluded from the hepatic artery and fed via the portal vein. Transarterial radioembolization (TARE), also called selective internal radiation therapy (SIRT), is a form of brachytherapy in which intra-arterially injected microspheres loaded with ^{90}Y serve as sealed sources for internal radiation purposes.[7,8]

There are two types of commercially available radioactive microspheres: one is made of glass (TheraSphere, MDS Nordion, Ottawa, Ontario, Canada) and the other resin (SIR-Spheres; Sirtex Medical Limited, Sydney, Australia), although they both use ^{90}Y as the radiation-emitting isotope. ^{90}Y is a pure β emitter with half-life of 64.2 hours (94% of the energy is emitted in the first 11 days) and average tissue penetration of 2.5 mm (isolation for radiation protection is not needed after implantation). Due to their small size (25–45 µm), microspheres produce no significant ischemic effect. To avoid misplacement of particles in extrahepatic territories, a thorough angiographic evaluation is performed 1 to 2 weeks prior to treatment to detect and eventually occlude aberrant vessels arising from hepatic arteries that may feed the gastrointestinal tract, and to measure the hepatopulmonary shunting using technetium-99 m-labeled macroaggregated albumin (^{99m}Tc-MAA). Patients can only be considered for TARE provided that their liver function is preserved (serum total bilirubin < 2 mg/dL) and they have no ascites or hepatic encephalopathy. TARE is generally well tolerated and a postembolization syndrome like the one that appears after transarterial chemoembolization is uncommon.

Attention has been paid to the intrinsic different activity distribution of resin and glass spheres at the microscopic scale, with dosimetric and radiobiologic consequences. Dedicated studies and mathematical models have been used to explore this issue and explain some clinical evidences, for example, the shift of dose to higher toxicity thresholds using glass as compared with resin spheres.[7]

RE represents a promising therapy for liver-predominant disease in patients with adequate functional liver reserve. For patients with a good performance status and sufficient liver reserve without other significant comorbidities, treatment could be considered either after the progression of liver metastases during treatment hiatus (after first-, second-, or nth-line chemotherapy), at an early line in tumors that respond poorly to chemotherapy (i.e., cholangiocarcinoma), or in treatment-refractory disease. Additional details on this therapy are included in a multidisciplinary consensus report covering many aspects of the procedure and patient selection, and provide level 2a medical evidence to support its use.[9]

RE is a proven treatment to slow disease progression and improve survival in patients with colorectal cancer liver metastases and hepatocellular carcinoma. Accumulating evidence supports its use in metastases from neuroendocrine tumors and breast cancer. Cancers with radiobiologic profiles similar to those of colorectal and breast cancer, including melanoma, lung cancer, and nodular cholangiocarcinoma, are being studied as candidates for RE. This treatment modality has also been shown to downsize hepatic tumors for potentially curative ablation in patients with breast, pancreatic, and colorectal cancer.

RE's efficacy appears to be independent of the primary tissue or cell of origin, and to result from high radiation doses to tumor alone. In an analysis of microdosimetry in four explanted livers from patients who were earlier treated with RE, Kennedy et al[10] noted that high numbers of microspheres were preferentially deposited in the periphery of tumors. Although cumulative radiation doses to the tumor ranged from 100 to more than 3,000 Gy, the normal liver showed little effect away from the tumors. Essentially, any vascular lesion with a favorable tumor-to-normal ratio of blood flow seems to respond well to this treatment modality. For instance, breast cancer has an α/β ratio (radiosensitivity coefficients for tumor type) similar to that of colorectal cancer, and studies have found that breast tumors are responsive to high-dose radiation regardless of their hormone receptor status, human epidermal growth factor 2 (HER2) status, or responsiveness to chemotherapy. The genetic composition of any given tumor, in a general sense, likely has a major influence on responsiveness to chemotherapy and radiation. It is therefore, appropriate to conclude that other tumors with radiobiologic profiles similar to colorectal and breast cancer will respond to RE in the liver.[9]

Multiple studies suggest that RE is effective in slowing disease progression and improving survival. To date, the recruitment of a large proportion of these patients for RE has been among those with advanced, chemorefractory disease. Recently, however, RE has been shown to downsize tumors for potentially curative surgical resection or ablation in patients with earlier unresectable primary or metastatic liver tumors that have received chemotherapy before or are chemorefractory.[11,12] In addition, unilobar RE has been reported to effect a radiation lobectomy in some patients, with improved tumor control even in patients who remain unresectable.[13–17]

The published clinical experience across many treatment centers also shows that the therapeutic ratio with RE compared with EBRT is significantly superior, and tumoricidal doses can be delivered with a relatively high safety margin. Therapeutic efficacy can be further improved by use of carefully chosen dosimetric techniques and meticulous treatment planning to mitigate serious complications.[8,18–20]

Radiation Effects in Normal Tissues

The therapeutic effect of external or internal radiotherapy necessitates exposure of normal tissues with significant radiation doses, and must thus be associated with an accepted rate of side effects.[21] Side effects from radiation have been well studied and are classified as acute, intermediate, or late effects.[22–25] Acute effects occur during a course of radiotherapy and are resolved within 4 weeks after the last treatment. Examples include epidermitis and mucositis due to injury to the skin and mucosal membranes, respectively. Intermediate effects are less common and occur within 8 to 12 weeks after ending radiation. An example is radiation pneumonitis, which reflects lung inflammation and is typically confined to the radiation portals. Late effects occur at least 9 months after the end of radiation and are usually the dose-limiting factor in clinical radiotherapy. Late effects include injury to specific tissues and organs within the radiation field or in the entrance or exit paths of the radiation beam. Other types of late effects due to irradiation include carcinogenesis (second tumors caused by radiation), teratogenesis (malformation of fetus, which occurs only rarely because pregnant women are almost never treated with radiation), and effects on growth and development stemming from irradiation in childhood.

The likelihood of developing a late effect depends on the total dose of radiation, the fraction size, the volume of tissue being treated, and concurrent treatments, such as chemotherapy. Late effects also depend upon prior or subsequent surgery, genetic factors unique to the individual patient, hypertension, age, pre-existing vascular damage, such as that from diabetes, and other pre-existing conditions (e.g., inflammatory bowel disease in patients who receive abdominal irradiation). The dose of radiation and/or volume of irradiated tissue is limited due to late effects, for example, tumors of the brain and spinal cord and locally advanced cancers of the lung, cervix, breast, and head and neck. Here, a selective normal tissue protector could allow a higher dose, a larger treatment volume, and/or reduced late normal tissue injury, thus increasing the therapeutic ratio.

In RE, millions of sources of radiation are liberated in the bloodstream. A simulation of the actual treatment is performed prior to RE by the injection of ^{99m}Tc-MAA particles, followed by planar and/or SPECT gamma-camera imaging. Several 3D software packages may take the distribution of ^{99m}Tc-MAA or ^{90}Y microspheres for a given patient and combine it with anatomic information (from CT or MRI) to yield absorbed dose estimates that are specific to that particular patient.[26] However, the absorbed dose to the liver or other organs cannot be directly measured in vivo after RE as it also occurs for other nuclear medicine procedures. Absorbed dose can be estimated from the data obtained during the preoperative simulation. With the Medical Internal Radiation Dose (MIRD) method of calculation, the dose absorbed by an organ from isotopes distributed homogeneously throughout that particular organ can be estimated. Using MIRD, much higher absorbed doses of radiation are tolerated after RE in comparison to EBRT.

As mentioned earlier, various clinical and mathematical models have been developed in the past two decades to understand and predict the risk of organ damage to radiation total doses, and dose per fraction schedules.[7] These NTCP models are based on observed complications after radiotherapy in a specific organ, with known daily and total dose data and specific clinical outcomes measured.[22,27] For hepatic radiation NTCP models, only external beam radiation with photons (not protons, carbon ions, ^{90}Y, or ^{131}I) has been explored. The most commonly accepted endpoint in hepatic NTCP models is radiation-induced liver disease (RILD), classically reported as TD5/5 and TD50/5. This translates into the total dose of photon radiation, typically to the whole liver, which creates a 5 and a 50% rate of RILD by 5 years post radiation, respectively.[28,29]

Using RT to treat cancer inevitably involves exposure of normal tissues. Consequently, patients may experience symptoms associated with normal tissue damage during the course of their therapy. These post-therapeutic effects may last for a few weeks or months to years later. Symptoms may be due to cell death or wound healing initiated within irradiated tissue, and may be precipitated by exposure to further injury or trauma. Many factors contribute to risk and severity of normal tissue reactions; these factors are site specific and vary according to time elapsed post treatment.[30]

Despite recent advances in radiation oncology aimed at making methodologies safer, it is not possible to exclude all normal tissues from the radiation field; and normal tissue damage remains a dose-limiting factor in the treatment of some tumor types (e.g., locally advanced cancers of the cervix, lung, head and neck, and brain).[31] A variety of effects to normal tissues from RT are discussed below.

Liver

The liver architecture consists of a parallel unit structure, with specific tolerance parameters regarding ionizing radiation. RT to liver tumors is limited by the relative radiosensitivity of the sinusoid endothelium, compared with significantly higher required doses of radiation to confidently destroy carcinoma cells.[32]

Acute and late effects of ionizing radiation to the liver have been described in the literature since the early 1960s.[33,34] During RT, acute or transient effects often are reported as elevation of liver enzymes, and depending on the treated volume, hematologic effects such as neutropenia and coagulopathy can occur. However, permanent effects can be produced, occurring weeks or months after radiation (late effects), such as fibrosis, persistent enzyme elevation, ascites, jaundice, and, rarely, RILD and fatal veno-occlusive disease (VOD).[35–38]

RILD is often referred to as *radiation hepatitis* and classically was described as occurring within 3 months of initiation of radiation, with rapid weight gain, increase in abdominal girth, liver enlargement, and, occasionally, ascites or jaundice, with elevation in serum alkaline phosphatase. The clinical picture resembled Budd–Chiari syndrome, but most patients survived, although some died of this condition without proven tumor progression. Descriptions illuminate that the whole liver could not be treated with radiation of more than 30 to 35 Gy in conventional fractionation (1.8–2 Gy/d, 5 d/wk) or else RILD or VOD was likely to occur.

Interestingly, VOD also can occur without RT in patients receiving high-dose chemotherapy in hematologic malignancies, alkaloids, toxic exposure to urethane, arsphenamine, and long-term oral contraceptives[39] as well as in patients receiving radiation combined with chemotherapy or radiation alone. The clinical presentation can differ between RILD and chemotherapy plus radiation liver disease, but the common pathologic lesion associated with RILD is VOD. The pathologic changes in VOD can affect a fraction of a lobe or the entire liver. It is best observed on low-power microscopy, which demonstrates severe congestion of the sinusoids in the central portion of the lobules with atrophy of the inner portion of the liver plates (zone 3).[37] Foci of yellow necrosis may appear in the center of affected areas. If the affected area is large, it can produce shrinkage and a wrinkled, granular capsule. The sublobular veins show significant obstruction by fine collagen fibers, which do not form in a larger vein (vena cava); this is a distinction between RILD and Budd–Chiari syndrome.[37,39] Most livers heal and display chronic changes after 6 months with little congestion but distorted lobular architecture with variable distances between central veins and portal areas. These chronic liver changes are typically asymptomatic but are reproducibly seen on liver biopsies as late as 6 years post presentation. Further investigation of the pathogenesis of VOD is difficult because most animals do not have VOD in response to radiation.[39]

References

1. Delaney G, Jacob S, Featherstone C, Barton M. The role of radiotherapy in cancer treatment: estimating optimal utilization from a review of evidence-based clinical guidelines. Cancer 2005;104(6):1129–1137

2. Harrison LB, Zietman AL. American society for radiation oncology intersociety summit summary. Int J Radiat Oncol Biol Phys 2010;76(3):643–648

3. Wallner PE, Anscher MS, Barker CA, et al. Current status and recommendations for the future of research, teaching, and testing in the biological sciences of radiation oncology: report of the American Society for Radiation Oncology Cancer Biology/Radiation Biology Task Force, executive summary. Int J Radiat Oncol Biol Phys 2014;88(1):11–17

4. Hall E. Radiobiology for the Radiologist. 5th ed. Philadelphia, PA: Lippincott Williams & Wilkins; 2000:5–16, 80–87

5. Christensen DM, Iddins CJ, Sugarman SL. Ionizing radiation injuries and illnesses. Emerg Med Clin North Am 2014;32(1):245–265

6. Kennedy AS, Raleigh JA, Perez GM, et al. Proliferation and hypoxia in human squamous cell carcinoma of the cervix: first report of combined immunohistochemical assays. Int J Radiat Oncol Biol Phys 1997;37(4):897–905

7. Cremonesi M, Chiesa C, Strigari L, et al. Radioembolization of hepatic lesions from a radiobiology and dosimetric perspective. Front Oncol 2014;4:210

8. Kennedy A, Nag S, Salem R, et al. Recommendations for radioembolization of hepatic malignancies using yttrium-90 microsphere brachytherapy: a consensus panel report from the radioembolization brachytherapy oncology consortium. Int J Radiat Oncol Biol Phys 2007;68(1):13–23

9. Coldwell D, Sangro B, Salem R, Wasan H, Kennedy A. Radioembolization in the treatment of unresectable liver tumors: experience across a range of primary cancers. Am J Clin Oncol 2012;35(2):167–177

10. Kennedy AS, Nutting C, Coldwell D, Gaiser J, Drachenberg C. Pathologic response and microdosimetry of (90)Y microspheres in man: review of four explanted whole livers. Int J Radiat Oncol Biol Phys 2004;60(5):1552–1563

11. Hoffmann RT, Jakobs TF, Kubisch CH, et al. Radiofrequency ablation after selective internal radiation therapy with yttrium-90 microspheres in metastatic liver disease-Is it feasible? Eur J Radiol 2010;74(1):199–205

12. Johnson DW, Mori KH, O'Laughlin SR, et al. Safety and efficacy of yttrium-90 labeled microsphere radiation treatment for hepatic metastases. Northeast Florida Med. 2009;60:37–41

13. Gaba RC, Bui JT, Knuttinen MG, Owens CA. Re: radiation lobectomy–a minimally invasive treatment model for liver cancer. J Vasc Interv Radiol 2009;20(10):1394–1396, author reply 1396

14. Gaba RC, Lewandowski RJ, Kulik LM, et al. Radiation lobectomy: preliminary findings of hepatic volumetric response to lobar yttrium-90 radioembolization. Ann Surg Oncol 2009;16(6):1587–1596

15. Gulec SA, Pennington K, Hall M, Fong Y. Preoperative Y-90 microsphere selective internal radiation treatment for tumor downsizing and future liver remnant recruitment: a novel approach to improving the safety of major hepatic resections. World J Surg Oncol 2009;7:6

16. Siddiqi NH, Devlin PM. Radiation lobectomy: a minimally invasive treatment model for liver cancer: case report. J Vasc Interv Radiol 2009;20(5):664–669

17. Vouche M, Lewandowski RJ, Atassi R, et al. Radiation lobectomy: time-dependent analysis of future liver remnant volume in unresectable liver cancer as a bridge to resection. J Hepatol 2013;59(5):1029–1036

18. Kennedy AS, McNeillie P, Dezarn WA, et al. Treatment parameters and outcome in 680 treatments of internal radiation with resin 90Y-microspheres for unresectable hepatic tumors. Int J Radiat Oncol Biol Phys 2009;74(5):1494–1500

19. Lewandowski RJ, Sato KT, Atassi B, et al. Radioembolization with 90Y microspheres: angiographic and technical considerations. Cardiovasc Intervent Radiol 2007;30(4):571–592

20. Murthy R, Brown DB, Salem R, et al. Gastrointestinal complications associated with hepatic arterial yttrium-90 microsphere therapy. J Vasc Interv Radiol 2007;18(4):553–561, quiz 562

21. Dörr W. Radiation effect in normal tissue: principles of damage and protection. Nucl Med (Stuttg) 2010;49(Suppl 1):S53–S58

22. Bentzen SM, Constine LS, Deasy JO, et al. Quantitative Analyses of Normal Tissue Effects in the Clinic (QUANTEC): an introduction to the scientific issues. Int J Radiat Oncol Biol Phys 2010;76(3, Suppl):S3–S9

23. Bentzen SM. Preventing or reducing late side effects of radiation therapy: radiobiology meets molecular pathology. Nat Rev Cancer 2006;6(9):702–713

24. Berkey FJ. Managing the adverse effects of radiation therapy. Am Fam Physician 2010;82(4):381–388, 394

25. Petersen C, Würschmidt F. Late Toxicity of radiotherapy: a problem or a challenge for the radiation oncologist? Breast Care (Basel) 2011;6(5):369–374

26. Flamen P, Vanderlinden B, Delatte P, et al. Multimodality imaging can predict the metabolic response of unresectable colorectal liver metastases to radio-embolization therapy with yttrium-90 labeled resin microspheres. Phys Med Biol 2008;53(22):6591–6603

27. Jackson A, Marks LB, Bentzen SM, et al. The lessons of QUANTEC: recommendations for reporting and gathering data on dose-volume dependencies of treatment outcome. Int J Radiat Oncol Biol Phys 2010; 76(3, Suppl):S155–S160

28. Dawson LA, Eccles C, Craig T. Individualized image guided iso-NTCP based liver cancer SBRT. Acta Oncol 2006;45(7):856–864

29. Dawson LA, Normolle D, Balter JM, McGinn CJ, Lawrence TS, Ten Haken RK. Analysis of radiation-induced liver disease using the Lyman NTCP model. Int J Radiat Oncol Biol Phys 2002;53(4):810–821

30. Stone HB, Coleman CN, Anscher MS, McBride WH. Effects of radiation on normal tissue: consequences and mechanisms. Lancet Oncol 2003;4(9):529–536

31. Rosen EM, Day R, Singh VK. New approaches to radiation protection. Front Oncol 2015;4:381

32. Klein J, Dawson LA. Hepatocellular carcinoma radiation therapy: review of evidence and future opportunities. Int J Radiat Oncol Biol Phys 2013;87(1):22–32

33. Ingold JA, Reed GB, Kaplan HS, Bagshaw MA. Radiation hepatitis. Am J Roentgenol Radium Ther Nucl Med 1965;93:200–208

34. Ogata K, Hizawa K, Yoshida M, et al. Hepatic injury following irradiation: a morphologic study. Tokushima J Exp Med 1963;10:240–251

35. Austin-Seymour MM, Chen GT, Castro JR, et al. Dose volume histogram analysis of liver radiation tolerance. Int J Radiat Oncol Biol Phys 1986;12(1):31–35

36. Dawson LA, Ten Haken RK, Lawrence TS. Partial irradiation of the liver. Semin Radiat Oncol 2001;11(3):240–246

37. Lawrence TS, Robertson JM, Anscher MS, Jirtle RL, Ensminger WD, Fajardo LF. Hepatic toxicity resulting from cancer treatment. Int J Radiat Oncol Biol Phys 1995;31(5):1237–1248

38. Lawrence TS, Ten Haken RK, Kessler ML, et al. The use of 3-D dose volume analysis to predict radiation hepatitis. Int J Radiat Oncol Biol Phys 1992;23(4):781–788

39. Fajardo LF, Berthrong M. Radiation Pathology REA. New York, NY: Oxford University Press; 2001

4 Interventional Radiology in the Treatment of the Cancer Patient

Douglas M. Coldwell

Introduction

Interventional radiology (IR) has a long history of being involved with cancer treatments. Visionary leaders in the field such as Sidney Wallace, MD, began the locoregional therapy of tumors and the use of image-guided therapy for diagnosis and treatment starting with the complications of the disease with obstruction of the biliary tree by pancreatic cancer, hemorrhage occurring from invasion into adjacent structures, to pulmonary emboli prophylaxis with inferior vena cava (IVC) filters. This naturally progressed to therapeutic options for primary and metastatic disease.

Local Tumor Diagnosis

Image-guided biopsy of masses began with fluoroscopically guided pulmonary biopsies. If the mass could be imaged and reliably identified on a chest radiograph, it is likely that it could be successfully biopsied with small-gauge needles, 20 to 22 gauge. Even hilar lesions could be biopsied, but the risks of hemorrhage and pneumothorax were far greater than peripheral lesions. A direct path to the lesion could be plotted using the rotational capabilities of the IR suite and the needle placed into the lesion with a confirmatory orthogonal view. The development of computed tomography (CT) guidance has allowed the precise biopsy of even smaller lesions than seen on fluoroscopy. A fine-needle aspirate should initially be obtained to determine if the lesion is at least suggestive of malignancy. The pathologist could then determine whether more tissue was needed. The availability of a pathologist on site when a biopsy is performed greatly enhances the likelihood of success. In fact, if the pathologist is not in or immediately outside the room, the interventional radiologist needs to insist that they be there. The positive biopsy rate will dramatically increase. Guiding needles slightly larger than the biopsy needle are usually placed so that multiple specimens may be obtained without the danger of repeatedly traversing the pleura. With the advent of genetic marker studies, the demand for larger biopsy specimens has rapidly increased. The use of core needles from 20 to 18 gauge has been helpful in providing these larger specimens. However, the larger the needle, the higher the risk of pneumothorax. Patients must be instructed to stop respiration as the needle is placed through the pleura to lessen the risk of a pneumothorax. However, even when all precautions are taken, the rate of pneumothorax occurring in any image-guided procedure is roughly 30%, of which about 1 in 10 or 3% of all biopsies require chest tube placement. If a pneumothorax is present, the needle should be aspirated as it is removed and much of the air present may be decompressed. Follow-up chest radiographs should be obtained in 1 and 4 hours to determine if the pneumothorax is enlarging. During this observation time, the patient must be admitted to a supervised holding area where they can be monitored for respiratory distress or decreased oxygen saturation and the interventional radiologist immediately available (**Fig. 4.1**). One of the basic tenets of IR becoming its own specialty must be that we should handle our own complications to the best of our ability and not have to rely on other services to do so. However, know our limitations and use consultations, for example, for cardiac clearance for chest pain by cardiology.

The ability and availability of equipment to place a chest tube must be present where lung biopsies are performed. Since there is little blood in the aspirated air, a simple Heimlich valve apparatus is usually sufficient and the patient is admitted overnight. A chest radiograph is obtained in the morning following admission and, if there is no sign of a pneumothorax, the valve is clamped for 4 hours and a repeat chest radiograph obtained. If there is still no pneumothorax, the tube may be safely removed. If the pneumothorax remains, the tube remains in place for another 12 to 24 hours and the above process repeated. Fortunately, most pneumothoraces resolve after the initial overnight admission. After 48 hours, a bronchopulmonary fistula should be considered and a consult to thoracic surgery made.

The other complication of pulmonary biopsy is hemorrhage. If large vascular structures are avoided and the possibility that the mass may be an arteriovenous malformation considered and excluded, significant hemorrhage is rare. The patient should be warned that small amounts of hemoptysis are expected, but large amounts are unusual and they should go to the nearest emergency room if it occurs. However, now that gene therapy is common, larger amounts of tissue are required for analysis with multiple core biopsies obtained. If numerous core biopsies are obtained, the patient should be watched for several hours for massive hemoptysis and warned that if it should occur, immediate admission to the emergency department is essential or bronchial artery embolization performed. If significant hemorrhage is noted on the CT, the patient should be placed in the decubitus position with the bleeding side down to assist in tamponading the bleed.

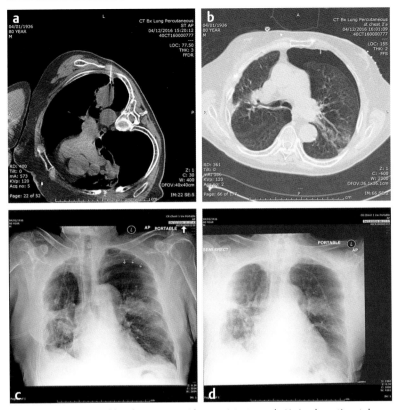

Fig. 4.1 An 80-year-old male presents with a persistent cough. He is a long-time tobacco user. **(a)** Computed tomography (CT) demonstrates needle in mass, which is pleural based. **(b)** CT demonstrates small pneumothorax occurring after biopsy. **(c)** Patient complained of pain in chest in holding area and difficulty breathing. An 8Fr pigtail catheter was placed. Chest radiograph demonstrates the catheter placed in pneumothorax, which is decompressed. Patient was admitted to the hospital overnight. **(d)** Chest radiograph 24 hours later does not show any evidence of pneumothorax.

Accuracy of needle biopsies varies by the number of passes made into the mass, the experience of the radiologist, and the availability of conscious sedation. With pathologists present to evaluate the specimens obtained, the accuracy is well over 90%. Occasionally, there will be patients who are unable to complete the biopsy even with conscious sedation and general anesthesia must be utilized. This is seen more frequently in pediatric patients and in patients with developmental and mental health issues. Obviously a good relationship with anesthesiology is a tremendous asset. Conversations with the anesthesiologists who cover "out of OR" (operating room) procedures will yield a better working relationship since they are very much out of their element and the necessary adjustments made to the room, the procedural sequence, and equipment availability can be made before the planned procedure and potential emergencies that arise during the procedure. Since general anesthesia usually requires that the patient be admitted to the postanesthesia care unit (PACU), the interventional radiologist should become familiar with the procedures and protocols there.

Once pulmonary biopsies became standard, the areas in which biopsies were requested blossomed to practically every portion of the body from the maxillary sinuses to the phalanges of the toes. This correlated with the growth of CT and ultrasound (US) technology that could produce images quickly. Many have used CT fluoroscopy, but objection to the increased radiation dose to both the patient and the physician has limited its routine utilization. Magnetic resonance imaging (MRI) guided biopsies require specialized nonmagnetic needles and equipment and may be limited to breast biopsies when no other imaging system will visualize the lesion. Additionally, the time required on the MRI is difficult to obtain since the biopsy takes longer than routine scans.

Local Tumor Therapy

From biopsies, the technology developed to ablate tumors. After all, if an interventional radiologist can place a needle into a lesion, isn't it a short jump to therapy? The initial tumor ablation processes were injection of ethanol or phenol into hepatic lesions. When ethanol comes into contact with cell walls, the walls rupture and the cell is almost instantaneously killed. The results varied since this is treatment of a single lesion with each placement of the needle. It is obviously not practical when numerous lesions are present, but when single inoperable lesions are present, ablative techniques should be considered. The use of ethanol or phenol directly injected into the tumor is unpredictable as to where the liquid travels and how much is enough. Most authors suggest that approximately one-third to one-half the volume of the tumor should be used. Larger lesions are not practical since the fluid may not reach the growing boundary of the tumor and collect inside the necrotic core and too much ethanol may also cause severe intoxication and poisoning. Its use should be limited to experienced physicians and be restricted to lesions that are less than 3 cm in diameter so that no more than approximately 10 to 15 mL of ethanol is utilized.[1]

In the early 1990s, the first radiofrequency ablation (RFA) units were produced and received Food and Drug Administration (FDA) clearance, which spurred the development of various array configurations and types of energy applied. RFA is the application of energy in the radiofrequency range (400–1,000 kHz) to a monopolar device so that the atoms within the tumor are either repelled or attracted by the charge on the device. Because the charge on the array is alternating at 60 Hz, the to-and-fro motion of the atoms causes heating due to interatomic friction. When the temperature rises above 46°C, irreversible damage is done to the area treated since the cell walls are disrupted and the cells desiccated. This is also reflected in the electrical resistance. Since the generators are of constant power, as the resistance to electrical current (or in the case of alternating current, the impedance) rises linearly, the current produced by the generator must fall by the square of the current so that the power is constant, producing the so-called "roll-off" of the current applied, shutting off the generator when the current reaches zero. A time–temperature relation exists such that if isolated thermocouples are placed in the tumor along with the array, heating them to a particular temperature for a specific time will give a treatment zone of a given diameter. This is in comparison to the bulk property of the constant power generator that is regulated by the resistance of the treated tumor. Both have their advocates, but the results are comparable. Since these are monopolar arrays, grounding pads must be used. Complications include the following:

- Incomplete heating and treatment of the tumor due to heat sink effects from nearby large blood vessels, bowel, organs.
- Hemorrhage due to the placement of the probe that is 14 gauge.
- Damage to adjacent organs or diaphragm.
- Seeding of the tumor along the probe tract (rare).
- Burns at the grounding pad site when the pads are not applied securely to the skin and are not observed during the procedure. Since the core body temperature may rise, sweating occurs and may cause the pads to become partially unattached, resulting in a high current density and a burn.

In the lung as in the liver, the largest tumors that can be treated with a very low recurrence rate measure 3 cm in diameter (**Fig. 4.2; Fig. 4.3**). Larger diameters increase the problems of recurrence since there may be incomplete or variable heating of the tumor even with larger arrays. A margin of at least 5 to 10 mm should be ablated around the tumor to assure that there is complete treatment. Smaller renal cell carcinomas (RCC) may also be treated with RFA. A useful technique is to inject very dilute contrast in the abdomen or retroperitoneum to move structures so that the tumor is accessible to treatment, so-called "hydrodissection" (**Fig. 4.4**). The same principles apply to microwave ablation, which is ablation utilizing a different portion of the electromagnetic spectrum. It is, however, faster than RFA, but the probes are larger in diameter and the equipment more expensive. If a larger tumor than the antennae on

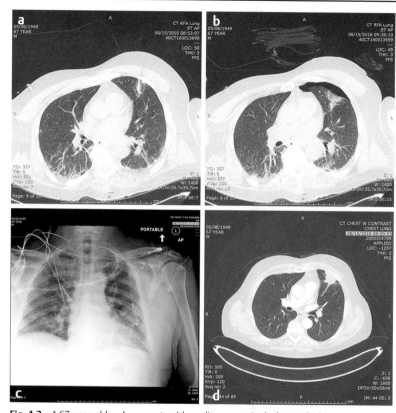

Fig. 4.2 A 67-year-old male presents with a solitary mass in the lung, which was a pancreatic carcinoma metastasis. **(a)** It was elected to treat this small mass with radiofrequency ablation (RFA). The 14-gauge coaxial needle is placed within the tumor and the tines extended. **(b)** The RFA was completed but a pneumothorax was present. **(c)** The patient began complaining of difficulty breathing on the computed tomography (CT) table and a 10Fr catheter placed into the pneumothorax via the third intercostal space in the mid-clavicular line and attached to a Heimlich valve. The patient was admitted overnight and the pneumothorax cleared in 24 hours. **(d)** A CT obtained 4 months later demonstrates the scarring that has occurred. The mass on positron emission tomography/CT was not avid for fluorodeoxyglucose, indicating this was scar formation.

the probe is treated, careful planning must be performed to overlap the fields to ensure that none of the tumor is untreated. This accounts for the higher recurrence rates in the larger tumors. A relatively recent addition to the ablative heating world was the bipolar probe to treat metastatic tumors in the spine and then follow the RFA with polymethyl methacrylate (PMMA) cement placement.

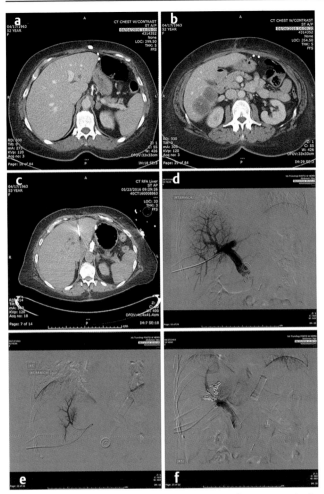

Fig. 4.3   A 52-year-old man presents with metastatic colon cancer to the liver only. The bulk of his disease is in the right lobe and a solitary mass in the left. **(a)** The computed tomography (CT) demonstrates the low attenuation mass in the left lobe of the liver, which represents the only site of disease in the left lobe. This was an enhanced CT scan. **(b)** Another slice from the same CT as in **(a)** demonstrates the large lesions in the right lobe. **(c)** The solitary left lobe mass is treated with radiofrequency ablation to be able to resect remaining disease in the right lobe. To do so, however, the left lobe must increase in size to compensate for the loss of normal liver tissue on the right. The residual liver must be at least 30% of the original size. **(d)** A transhepatic portal venogram is performed and demonstrates the flow to both sides of the liver. To enlarge the left lobe, the right lobe portal venous radicles need to be embolized with particles and coils. **(e)** A segmental portal vein radical in the right lobe that was embolized. **(f)** The final portal venogram demonstrating complete embolization of the right portal venous radicles with flow remaining to the left. The right hepatectomy was completed and the patient recovered without incident.

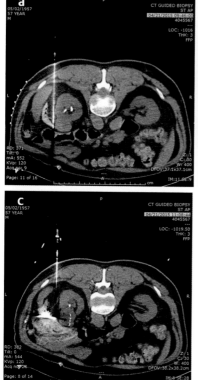
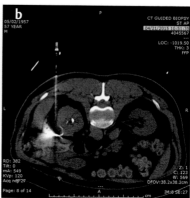

Fig. 4.4 A 57-year-old man presents with a mass on his left kidney that was renal cell carcinoma. **(a)** A needle is placed adjacent to the kidney and contrast and saline mixture injected to "hydrodissect" the kidney away from the spleen and allow placement of the radiofrequency ablation (RFA) coaxial needle. **(b)** The hydrodissection continues and the RFA needle is seen to be in the mass with the tines extended. **(c)** The RFA is completed as seen by the areas of gas within the tumor. The tumor eventually shrunk and scarred to a fluid containing structure. No nephrectomy was necessary.

Similarly, the use of cryotherapy to treat tumors was instituted in the late 1980s. This procedure requires the placement of multiple probes through which helium gas under pressure flows. A small chamber at the end of each needle allows the helium to expand and, according to the ideal gas law, the temperature is lowered significantly to well below –100°C, forming an ice ball at the tip of the probe. With multiple probes, the contour of this ice ball can be contoured to the shape of the tumor. This has been utilized with over 90% success in the treatment of renal as well as prostate, lung, bone, and soft-tissue tumors that are 4 cm or less in diameter. While it was used surgically in the liver, the large ice ball could shatter resulting in exsanguination of the patient. The percutaneous use of cryotherapy has been limited in the liver due to the surgical experience. The ice balls may be monitored by CT, US, or MRI imaging. The limitations to the treatment are that it is local and treats one tumor at a time (like RFA), takes somewhat longer than RFA or microwave therapy, and the equipment costs are higher than RFA. However, the results in the kidney and bone show promise.[2,3]

A new ablative instrument, irreversible electroporation (IRE) has been introduced. This, like so many other ablative techniques, began in the OR with its use in nonoperative tumors. It consists of multiple probes placed around the periphery of the tumor and electrical current of high voltage and low-amperage direct current are delivered between each pair of probes. This is performed under general anesthesia with cardiac gating so that the electrical current is not placed during a sensitive portion of the cardiac cycle. When the tumor cell is treated, the pores in the cell wall remain open and the differential osmolarity between the inside and outside of the cell is eliminated and the cell undergoes apoptosis.[4] For advanced pancreatic primaries, IRE appears to increase overall survival and progression-free survival.[5] IRE has been touted as not being sensitive to the heat sink effect of RFA and being safe for surrounding blood vessels; however, recent articles have noted that the vascular complication rate is near 50% and the effectiveness about the same as RFA for hepatic tumors.[6] The difference between RFA and IRE is the large investment to obtain the equipment, the high cost of the probes, and the extended time required placing the probes precisely under CT guidance.

Venous Access Devices

Probably the most performed procedure in IR today is the placement of venous access devices. It is also the one procedure that links the medical oncologist to IR and forms the basis of a close working and referral relationship. Those practices that have an easy referral system in place will also be able to transform that relationship to the performance of more aggressive and advanced cancer therapy protocols. The skill of the interventional radiologist performing the device placement is also a measure on which the relationship is built. Adherence to the principles of sterile procedures is an absolute necessity since the patients may have these lines for weeks to years. Additionally, the number of central line infections has been a benchmark on which the Centers for Medicare & Medicaid Services grades, judges, and rewards or penalizes the hospital through their reimbursement of services.

Basic laboratory results should be obtained so that coagulation times, platelet count, and the potential for ongoing infections can be evaluated to minimize the risk to the patient. Removing a device recently placed due to infection or a large hematoma arising is inexcusable when the laboratory results can lead to appropriate patient selection and good surgical technique can avoid untoward results. Since there are essentially four to six placement sites available for long-term access device placement, removal of a device and losing one of these sites is a potentially catastrophic problem.

The tunneled central line (the Hickman catheter) was the first to be approved in the 1980s and was almost universally placed in the OR by surgeons. The traditional surgical method of placement of these lines involved a blind puncture of the lateral portion of the left (usually) subclavian vein after local anesthesia and placement of a wire into the superior vena cava (SVC) followed by placement of local anesthesia of a tract in the anterior chest wall that is at least 10-cm long. The catheter is then brought through this tunnel by using a tapered metal tunneler and exits at the venotomy site. A "peel-away" sheath is then placed into the vein and the catheter placed into the venous system as the sheath is torn and removed leaving the outer ends of the catheter outside of the patient's chest and the tip in the SVC. This placement is then confirmed by a chest radiograph or under fluoroscopy. Surprisingly enough, the acceptable position of the tip of the catheter has been described as essentially anywhere in the SVC as long as blood could be aspirated. Unfortunately, this process included placement of the tip against the right lateral SVC wall where infusions of chemotherapy cannot only cause a fibrin sheath at the tip but a pseudoaneurysm to form in the SVC (**Fig. 4.5**). The misplacement of the catheter

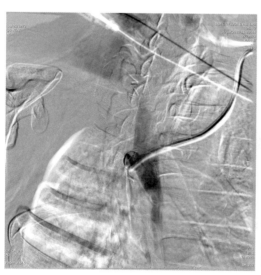

Fig. 4.5 A 62-year-old female presents with a malfunctioning subcutaneous port. Injection of contrast through the port demonstrates that it was placed by a subclavian puncture and the tip was against the right lateral wall of the superior vena cava (SVC). It had been utilized for chemotherapy for 2 months. There is a pseudoaneurysm of the SVC at the point where the catheter came into contact. This complication only happens when a subclavian approach is utilized and the catheter placed by "feel" and a chest radiograph obtained afterward to detect a pneumothorax.

is not the only risk entailed by placing the catheter through a subclavian venous puncture. Others include compression of the catheter so that it "pinches off" through the action of the shoulder muscles and ligaments and eventually results in a broken catheter in the right atrium or pulmonary artery (**Fig. 4.6**). These catheters are then retrieved by IR, but they are barely visible under fluoroscopy and are difficult to snare with a retrieval device. If they have been present for weeks to months, it is likely they are attached to the endothelium of the heart and the SVC, making the catheter impossible to retrieve. If the catheter is causing arrhythmias or thrombi to form, it must then be removed surgically. The blind puncture of the subclavian vein also brings the risk of pneumothorax, and older sheaths utilized to place the catheter in the venous system risked air emboli since

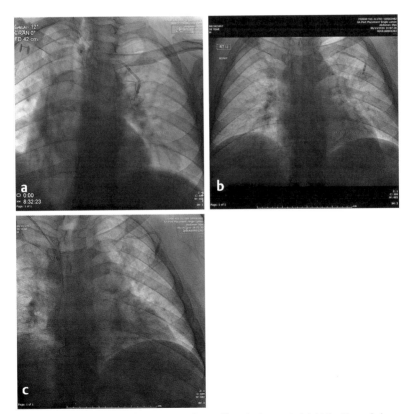

Fig. 4.6   A 57-year-old male presents with a malfunctioning port. **(a)** At the time of placement, a slight jog in the course of the catheter under the clavicle indicates that this catheter is pinched and will eventually break. **(b)** Six months later, the catheter is fractured and the distal end is in the right atrium. **(c)** A snare is introduced and the fragment removed.

they did not have a diaphragm at the end to prevent the entrance of air. While air emboli can still rarely occur, the interventional radiologist must be familiar with the treatment: place the patient in the left lateral decubitus position and wait until the air dissipates. If the patient is left in the supine position, it is possible that a large air bolus may cause "vapor lock" in the pulmonary artery with dire consequences.

More modern techniques are utilized in the IR suite where, under US guidance, the jugular vein is punctured and a wire placed into the right atrium or inferior vena cava (IVC). This approach avoids the potential "pinch off" from the subclavian approach and the possibility of a pneumothorax. A tunnel is then anesthetized along the chest wall and the catheter brought from the chest to the venotomy site. A diaphragm-containing peel-away sheath is then placed and the catheter placed in the inferior portion of the SVC or the superior portion of the right atrium under fluoroscopic control. The risks from this approach are significantly less and the likelihood of a successful placement is increased. It has also been demonstrated that the results of the jugular approach are superior to the subclavian in duration of patency, infection rate, and complications.[7]

The long-term problems with tunneled central lines include the formation of fibrin sheaths at the tip (**Fig. 4.7**), which can be removed by using a bolus of tissue plasminogen Activator, fibrin stripping by using a retrieval snare and sliding it along the catheter, or, finally, exchange of the catheter by placement of two wires through the lumens, removing the catheter and placement of a new catheter through the same tract. If the tract becomes infected, it may be treated with antibiotics if the organism is not a gram-negative species or the patient has leukemia or lymphoma, saving the venous access site.[8]

If a catheter is in place for months, it is not uncommon to see central venous stenoses that limit the flow through the catheter and can cause upper extremity edema. These narrowings should be addressed by balloon angioplasty. Since these stenoses are long standing and in the venous system, they have a high fibrin content, while the arterial stenoses are usually due to atherosclerotic disease. It is common to angioplasty these stents and the balloon may have to be inflated for up to 3 minutes. The use of stents is common to treat these stenoses. Uncovered stents are usually utilized so as not to block any small venous inflow (**Fig. 4.8**).

Implanted Ports

Placement of implantable ports is but a small step beyond the placement of tunneled catheters. A small pocket is made under the selected clavicle just slightly larger than the port to be utilized. A single incision is made and blunt dissection is performed. The catheter may be cut to length and

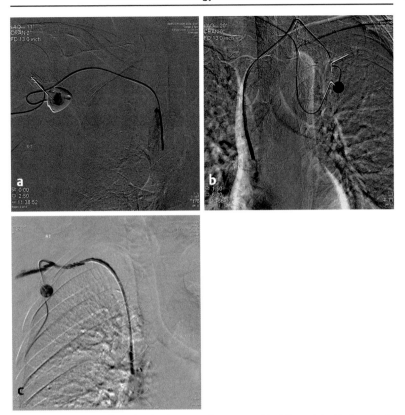

Fig. 4.7 Examples of fibrin sheaths that typically present with ability to inject but unable to aspirate the port. **(a)** Mild sheath at the tip that shows contrast exiting into the superior vena cava approximately 2 cm superior to the end of the catheter. **(b)** More severe fibrin sheath that extends from the tip proximally about half the length of the catheter. **(c)** Severe sheath that extends almost to the puncture site and exits into the subclavian vein.

placed before attachment to the reservoir, but most prefer to attach them before placing the catheter into the venous system to prevent air emboli. If the pocket around the port is tight enough, it is unnecessary to place any sutures; however, if a generous pocket is made, suturing the port to the backside of the pocket insures that the port will not rotate and make the access impossible. Ports have been placed and utilized for several years. When removing such long-term ports, it is sometimes extremely difficult when calcification occurs around the catheter and a thick rind of scar tissue envelops the port. Placement of the tip of the catheter is the same for tunneled lines. Ports should be placed within the chest tissue taking

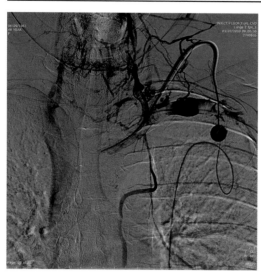

Fig. 4.8 A 48-year-old patient presents with a malfunctioning port. The injection of contrast through the port demonstrates that the left brachiocephalic vein is occluded and there are multiple collateral veins present. This is far more common in subclavian venous punctures. The occlusion may be crossed and dilated with a stent, but a thrombolytic agent may be necessary to clear the recent clot.

into account the amount of breast tissue present so that when the patient stands, the catheter does not automatically withdraw to an unusually high position where it cannot be used successfully. This can be done by pressing the breast tissue inferiorly when the pocket site is selected. Placement of the port in the axilla or deeper than 5 mm beneath the skin surface should be avoided as it inhibits the access of the port. In patients receiving radiation therapy to the chest, the port should be placed on the opposite side to where the radiation is being administered since the port can deflect the photons and influence the dose to the tumor.

There has been a movement to place more peripherally inserted central catheters (PICCs) in the extremities, most commonly for long-term antibiotics but also for chemotherapy. US placement involves the selection of an extremity vein (with or without placement of a tourniquet so that the vein will be enlarged), usually the brachial or basilic. The skin is then anesthetized and the vein entered with a 21-gauge needle, followed by placement of a 0.018-inch wire into the vein. The venotomy site is preferably above the elbow and attention should be paid to the potential for the needle to pass through a nerve; if the patient complains of pain radiation down the extremity, another site should be selected. The skin site is then dilated with a 4- to 6-Fr dilator and a measurement wire placed to the inferior SVC and the length noted. The PICC is then cut to this length and inserted through a small peel-away sheath and secured to the skin.

While extremity veins are usually selected for PICC placement, the lines can be placed in almost any venous structure that is:

- Close to the skin.
- Visible by US.
- Is large enough to accept the catheter without it occluding.
- The tip can be placed into a central vein.

For example, the inferior epigastric vein, which travels along the abdominal wall, can be utilized for access. Preservation of venous access sites is essential in the treatment of any patient as there are only a handful, the internal/external jugular, subclavian (not preferred), femoral, and directly into the IVC immediately superior to the pelvic brim. The latter is a last resort since it requires direct puncture into the IVC and tunneling through the soft tissues of the flank. The femoral venous access is also not preferred due to the difficulty in managing the sterility or cleanliness of the site. There are often more central line infections when the femoral vein is utilized.

A new variation of the PICC line is the tunneled PICC, which is inserted in the jugular vein and tunneled inferiorly similar to any other tunneled line. These lines are 6 Fr in diameter, double lumen, and placed centrally. These have been used more frequently in a patient who is not on dialysis currently but is expected to be placed on it imminently. This type of central line spares the veins of the extremities so that they can be used for dialysis shunts/grafts.

All tunneled lines have a Dacron cuff in the portion that is passed through the tunnel so that the skin can grow into it and secure it. This occurs 3 to 4 weeks after placement so that the skin sutures are not as important in these longer-term lines. This, however, affects their removal, as blunt dissection along the catheter track is necessary to easily remove them. Sometimes, the catheter is removed and leaves the Dacron cuff within the soft tissues. To remove it, it requires a cutdown and exposure with its removal. Usually these cuffs are left in place, but the patient must be told about it so that if they feel a small lump they know what it is. Mammography will detect these cuffs and, without the information and documentation that they are the residua of a tunneled line, may be mistaken for a malignancy.

Nontunneled central lines are placed in a similar fashion without the necessity of a tunnel. These are utilized when the patient is an in-patient and removed before their discharge. Adequate suturing is necessary to avoid displacement of the line.

Interventional Therapies

The first embolotherapy requests were likely for controlling bleeding from tumor invasion into adjacent structures. This requires superselective catheterization and led, eventually, to the development of the microcatheter and 0.018-inch and smaller diameter guide wires. Hypervascular tumors such as sarcomas, renal cell carcinomas (RCC), hepatomas, and melanomas invade adjacent organs such as the pancreas, kidney, or duodenum and cause hemorrhage that can be life-threatening. While coil embolization of the vessel causing the hemorrhage may or may not be sufficient to halt it, other embolic agents need to be considered and individualized for every patient. The choice of embolic agent is critical since the use of particulates to embolize bleeding should only be utilized when there are no normal tissues downstream to infarct. For example, the invasion into the duodenum of pancreatic carcinoma usually requires the placement of 5- to 6-mm-diameter platinum coils into the proximal and distal gastroduodenal artery (GDA). If particles are utilized, the pancreatic head will be embolized, resulting in at least pancreatitis, pseudocyst, or necrosis (**Fig. 4.9**).

Embolotherapy

Patients most likely to benefit from directed therapy to treat hemorrhage from a tumor are those in whom the tumor mass can be separated on angiography from normal tissues. Embolization of normal tissues may be necessary to halt the bleeding, but it is important to recognize the collaterals that form to feed the normal embolized tissues. To perform embolotherapy correctly and safely, the choice of embolic agent is the first critical decision to be made after accepting the referral. This choice begins with the decision of whether they are to be permanent, semipermanent, or temporary. Permanent embolic agents include coils or vascular plugs made of nitinol. Each of these is available in a range of sizes that will allow most vessels to be embolized in a few minutes after placing the catheter. Placement of a microcatheter is easier than a 5-Fr catheter and the microcoils are effective since they are not only made of platinum, but also have Dacron fibers interwoven into them that promote platelet aggregation and thrombus formation. Other permanent agents include ethanol, Sotradecol (which contains ~45% ethanol), or glue. These are more liquid agents and must be treated with extreme care since they can penetrate deeply into the small arterioles and cause necrosis. Ethanol is immediately toxic to the endothelial lining of arteries, causing this lining to slough and exposing the media, which is thrombogenic. When using ethanol, complete tissue destruction downstream from the catheter tip is expected and argues for meticulous catheter

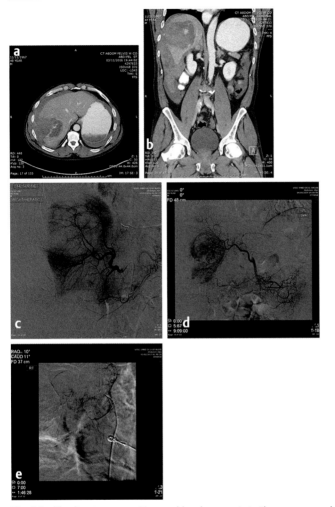

Fig. 4.9 Bleeding tumors: a 48-year-old male presents to the emergency department. He is hypotensive with a falling hematocrit without significant trauma. A computed tomography scan is obtained. **(a)** Axial scan demonstrates a cirrhotic liver with the hepatocellular carcinoma hemorrhaging. **(b)** Coronal reconstruction demonstrates that a large mass in the right lobe of the liver is hemorrhaging into the peritoneum. **(c)** An arteriogram of the liver shows that the arteries in the right lobe are stretched and draped around the large hematoma. Even though there was no specific bleeding site identified, this artery was embolized with 100-μ diameter particles until stasis. At that point, his hypotension resolved. **(d)** A hepatic arteriogram of another patient whose hepatocellular carcinoma was demonstrated to have a bleeding site and was embolized with particulates. **(e)** A bronchial arteriogram readily shows the tumor vascularity that caused the patient hemoptysis. This was embolized with 100-μ diameter particles and care was taken not to embolize the anterior spinal artery.

placement. The amount of ethanol to use is estimated by seeing the penetration into the tissues by contrast. The use of a balloon occlusion catheter may be of assistance when using alcohol, but it should be well aspirated before the balloon is deflated so that the products of the embolization are not refluxed into a neighboring artery causing embolization to areas that are not intended. For example, ethanol has been utilized for the embolization of RCC prior to nephrectomy so that the devascularized tissues will not cause extraordinary blood loss due to the hypervascular nature of the RCC. The use of an occlusion balloon has been promoted thinking that the balloon will keep the debris and alcohol contained. However, if this catheter is not completely and well aspirated and flushed and re-aspirated after the ethanol use, some ethanol and debris can be, and has been reported to have, refluxed into the superior mesenteric artery. Others have foregone the use of the occlusion balloon arguing that the blood flow is necessary to carry the ethanol into the distal arterioles to have a more complete embolization.

Glue, another permanent agent, presents its own set of peculiarities, problems, and demands. Catheters must be flushed with D5W before injecting the glue through a glass syringe that is used to aspirate the glue from a glass container. The glue should not come into contact with plastic syringes or an ionic solution until it arrives in the blood stream as either causes it to begin polymerization. The glue itself is not radio-opaque but, when mixed with the enclosed tantalum powder, becomes easily visualized under fluoroscopy. When the flow is fast and distal embolization is desired, a more liquid and delayed polymerization is used by adding Pantopaque or Ethiodol to the mixture. If more proximal obstruction is desired, the less the polymerization is delayed. However, the sooner the polymerization begins, the more likely the catheter can be permanently glued in place if not removed as the last bit of glue is placed. There are catheters in the market that can retard the attachment of the glue so that the likelihood of being glued to the artery is now significantly less. Some of the gluelike agents will also not cling to the catheter as well as the NBCA (*n*-Butyl cyanoacrylate) glue. The permanent liquid agents are usually used in the setting of arteriovenous malformation treatment and less so in tumor or hemorrhage.

While many consider particles to be permanent, they are actually a semipermanent agent since, over time, they are incorporated into the vascular wall and flow may be re-established. This may occur over days to weeks so that the tumor distal to the embolization site may have become necrotic. The size of the particle is a key determinant to how fast the recanalization occurs. The larger the particle, the more proximal the occlusion, meaning collaterals are more likely to quickly form as these vessels are larger, more available, and more numerous. The smaller the particle, the more distal it occludes the artery, and necrosis of tissue may ensue. A general rule of thumb for selection of size of particle is that if the artery in which the catheter is placed feeds only tumor, it is safe to use the 40-μ-diameter particles, the smallest particles currently available. However, if this particle size is utilized and normal tissue is embolized, there will be normal tissue necrosis with islands of viable tumor present. If normal tissues must be sacrificed when embolizing, larger particles, 100 to 300 µ in diameter, can be used. Larger particles than these cause collateral formation almost instantaneously.

A relative contraindication to embolotherapy of tumor in the liver is occlusion of the portal vein. Conventional wisdom has it that, by occluding the hepatic artery, all flow to the liver will be lost and necrosis of the lobe will occur. This is rarely the case, as the intrahepatic arterial collaterals will open quickly and supply the embolized lobe as long as the smallest agents are not utilized. If a lobe of liver has been completely replaced by tumor, and, in cases of hepatocellular carcinoma (HCC), for example, the portal vein is invaded or occluded by tumor, there has been a fair amount of hesitation to using embolotherapy because of the risk of necrosing the entire lobe. However, if the tumor has completely or nearly completely replaced the lobe, the only tissue that will necrose is tumor. In such a case, the smallest embolic agent available, 40-µ-diameter particles, can be used to insure that the tumor is thoroughly treated.

Chemoembolization has changed from its original design of a slurry of Ethiodol or lipiodol, both iodinated poppy seed oils, with a chemotherapy agent. The oil is phagocytized into the cancer cell bringing the emulsified chemotherapy agent with it as was demonstrated by making autoradiographs of ^{131}I-lipiodol.[9] The chemotherapy agents utilized in these treatments include Adriamycin, cisplatin, mitomycin C, or irinotecan, individually or in combination. While such "traditional" chemoembolization showed promise as a treatment for metastatic tumor in the liver, it was especially operator dependent to insure the optimal chemotherapeutic concentration and emulsification since the lipiodol actually dissolved the polycarbonate three-way stopcocks that were used to emulsify the oil and chemotherapy agent. Additionally, the commercial availability of the lipiodol/Ethiodol has been sporadic. After the emulsion had been administered, the hepatic arteries were embolized with particles until stasis of flow occurred. The exact definition of "stasis" is problematical since this is another operator-specific variable.

These problems have been somewhat circumvented by the use of drug-eluting beads that are soaked in either Adriamycin or irinotecan for a specified period to obtain maximal concentration and then the tumor is embolized with a specific dose of the bead–chemotherapy combination and may or may not be embolized to stasis after the delivery of the chemotherapy-loaded beads. Unlike the original chemoembolization, the cells are bathed in the chemotherapy until the dose has become depleted without a mechanism to insure that the chemotherapy will actually get into the cell itself. Additional problems with this type of chemotherapy include the use of irinotecan, a mildly effective chemotherapy agent on its own, but when used systemically, the effectiveness is related to the conversion of irinotecan to SN-38 by an enzyme occurring in normal liver but not in tumors. SN-38 is 1,000 times as effective as the irinotecan. Because of the sclerotic nature of irinotecan, patients report significant pain, above and beyond the postembolization pain. The exposure of the tumors to a high dose of either irinotecan or Adriamycin for a few hours when neither are very effective chemotherapy agents in the tumors in which they are used systemically (irinotecan – 15% in metastatic colorectal cancer and Adriamycin – 18% in HCC when used as single agents) has led to questioning of the rationale of this type of chemoembolization. Potentially, the chemotherapeutic agents are merely sclerotic agents and extend the range of the embolotherapy to smaller vessels. Research is beginning to determine the mechanism of action of the chemotherapy drug used in the drug-eluting beads. Nevertheless, response to this therapy has been reported to be in the range of 50% in HCC and 40% in metastatic colorectal cancer to the liver, which is not significantly different from bland embolization.[10] Bland embolization of tumors has also been utilized to enhance the effect of RFA treatment of liver and renal tumors[11] (**Fig. 4.10**).

Radioembolization

The newest embolotherapy agent is radioactive particles using ^{90}Y either as a constituent of the glass bead or adherent to the surface of resin beads. Both agents are of similar size, 35 to 40 µ in diameter, but the glass particle has a higher activity per particle of 2,500 Bq in comparison to the resin at 50 Bq per particle, which requires the resin bead to use more particles to treat the tumor than the former to obtain the same activity administered to the tumor. Both beads are designed to treat the tumor with at least 150 Gy while exposing the liver to less than 50 Gy, the dose at which radiation-induced liver disease (RILD) is expected.

As expected, the more vascular the tumor, the better the outcome with yttrium or any of the embolotherapy agents. HCC, intrahepatic cholangiocarcinoma, renal cell carcinoma, and metastatic neuroendocrine tumors respond extremely well. Even moderately vascular tumors such as colorectal carcinoma, ovarian carcinoma metastases, and breast cancer respond well. A retrospective study of over 600 patients with colorectal cancer determined that there was a 96% response rate with the median survival after yttrium therapy of about a year (**Fig. 4.11**).

The data on the frequency and treatment of RILD have been extrapolated from the radiation therapy literature that measures its prevalence in external beam treatments to the liver. Recently, the idea that RILD due to radioembolization may be a specific subset of RILD since the radiation is brachytherapy and the symptoms usually appear before 90 days after

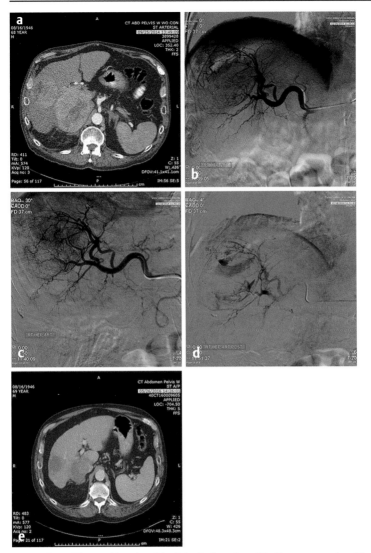

Fig. 4.10 A 69-year-old male with cirrhosis from hepatitis C now presents with upper abdominal discomfort. **(a)** Computed tomography (CT) with contrast demonstrates two hypervascular masses within the liver. **(b)** The initial arteriogram demonstrates the extreme hypervascularity of the lesion. Transarterial chemoembolization (TACE) was then performed using 100- to 300-μ beads loaded with 150-mg doxorubicin. **(c)** Midway through the injection, this arteriogram shows the partial filling of the tumor. **(d)** At the end of the embolization, contrast stasis is noted with in the tumor. **(e)** After two TACE treatments, this CT was obtained showing no enhancement around the lesions that are now noticeably decreased in size.

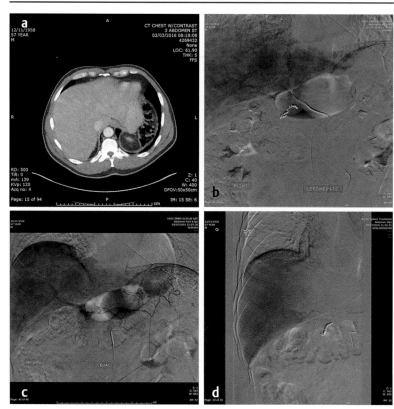

Fig. 4.11 A 57-year-old woman with metastatic neuroendocrine tumor presented with uncontrollable diarrhea that kept her at home and dehydrated. (**a**) The computed tomography scan does not fully appreciate the amount of tumor present as it was isointense with the hepatic parenchyma. Her chromogranin A level at this time was 3,500. (**b**) On her screening arteriogram, the diffuse nature of the small milliary tumors is noted on the celiac arteriogram. (**c**) Complete replacement of the left lobe of the liver is noted on this left hepatic arteriogram. It was elected to treat the majority of the disease first, that is, the right lobe, then bring her back for a second treatment on the left. (**d**) At the time of the second treatment, this right hepatic arteriogram was performed and demonstrates no evidence of any tumor blush in the right lobe. Her diarrhea had significantly slowed and her chromogranin A level had dropped to 900. After her second treatment, the diarrhea resolved completely and she is well palliated with a chromogranin A level of less than 50.

treatment with a larger rise in the liver function tests than usually seen in RILD, jaundice, ascites, and increased bilirubin levels without dilated biliary ducts. Biopsy results demonstrate sinusoidal congestion around the perivenule areas, hepatic atrophy, and necrosis around the central veins with formation of thrombus. This is consistent with veno-occlusive disease (VOD). Consequently, this has become known as radioembolization-induced liver disease (REILD) and is usually treated with high-dose steroids and occasionally Trental, which hopefully will preclude the formation of widespread VOD in the liver. In serious cases of REILD, a transjugular intrahepatic portosystemic shunt has been demonstrated to help reverse the liver function decline.[12]

Resin beads have also reported to be more embolic than the glass. However, this may not necessarily be a bad characteristic since the tumors are usually hypervascular and will respond to embolization alone. The major objection to this embolic effect is that the tumors are completely ischemic and, without the available oxygen to enhance radical formation to multiply the effect on tumor DNA (deoxyribonucleic acid), such a treatment would be less effective. Since tumors regrow in areas that have been embolized with particles only to stasis, it appears that no tumor is completely without oxygen and the idea that such a treatment is less effective is not confirmed by the published data. Such embolization may actually be therapeutic since bland embolization is an option for treatment. Investigators have also utilized nonradioactive beads to embolize the liver of a pig and noted that no significant embolization or stasis of flow occurred at normal numbers of particles administered. Stasis occurring during administration of radioactive beads is likely due to an incorrect dose, prior bevacizumab therapy with reduction of the tumoral vascular volume, or an incorrect estimation of the tumor volume.

Inclusion criteria for radioembolization include the following:

- Adults.
- Liver dominant but not necessarily exclusive disease.
- Serum total bilirubin less than 2 mg/dL. If a patient has a bilirubin level greater than this, the likelihood of liver failure is increased.

Exclusion criteria include the following:

- Greater than 70% of the liver replaced by tumor.
- Serum bilirubin greater than 2 mg/dL.
- Hepatic artery to hepatic vein shunting so that greater than 10% (for glass beads) or 20% (for resin beads) is shunted to the pulmonary circulation.
- Liver failure.
- Ascites.
- Hepatic encephalopathy.

The shunt to the pulmonary circulation is particularly important as such a shunt can induce radiation pneumonitis. Radiation pneumonitis has a typical "bat wing" appearance on CT and is treated with high-dose steroids. Fortunately, this is a very rare complication. Both products mandate a check for this shunt by performing an injection of [99mTc] labeled macroaggregated albumin (MAA) spheres at the treatment position for the catheter and then performing a planar or single-photon emission computed tomography (SPECT) scan in Nuclear Medicine so that the exact shunting can be calculated. This is performed at an initial screening arteriogram.

This screening arteriogram is also necessary to determine the arterial anatomy of the upper abdomen, since only 55% of patients have "normal" arterial anatomy. The differing types of celiac origin variants are given in **Table 4.1**. Not only are the celiac trunks variable, but also the arterial supply to the liver can be variable. The most common variants are given in **Table 4.2**.

If the left hepatic artery originates from the left gastric artery, when the left lobe is treated with radioembolization, particles may reflux into the gastric arteries causing an ulcer. The left hepatic artery may be embolized with a coil allowing the intrahepatic collateral vessels to enlarge and enable the treatment of the left lobe from infusion into the right hepatic artery. If the tumor burden is large and the patient has had bevacizumab, the postembolization syndrome may result (**Fig. 4.12**). At this screening study, embolization of any arteries that may carry refluxed particles to the stomach (notably the right gastric artery and an accessory left gastric artery originating from the left hepatic artery) or pancreas (GDA) is performed. Questions have been raised about the utility of the GDA embolization if the artery is well away from the site of the introduction of the ^{90}Y beads, the manufacturers' recommendations still suggest this embolization and, given the potential of radiation-induced ulcers in the duodenum and pancreatitis, this procedure should still be performed. The advent of a partially occluding catheter during the introduction of the ^{90}Y beads seems to be of assistance,

Table 4.1 Anatomical variants of the celiac axis

Type	Description
I	Classic celiac trunk
II	Hepatosplenic trunk
III	Hepatogastric trunk
IV	Hepatosplenic, mesenteric trunk
V	Gastrosplenic trunk
VI	Celiac–mesenteric trunk
VII	Celiac–colic trunk
VIII	No celiac trunk

Table 4.2   Hepatic arterial normal variants

Type	Description
I	Normal anatomy
II	Replaced left hepatic artery originating from the left gastric artery
III	Replaced right hepatic artery originating from the superior mesenteric artery
IV	Coexistence of types II and III
V	Accessory left hepatic artery originating from the left gastric artery
VI	Accessory right hepatic artery originating from the superior mesenteric artery
VII	Accessory left hepatic artery originating from the left gastric artery and accessory right hepatic artery originating from the superior mesenteric artery
VIII	Accessory left hepatic artery originating from the left gastric artery and replaced right hepatic artery originating from the superior mesenteric artery
IX	Common hepatic artery originating from the superior mesenteric artery
X	Right and left hepatic arteries originating from the left gastric artery

but the flow dynamics of the hepatic arteries are disturbed and the beads appear to be delivered in more of a bolus that is carried by a pulse of blood rather than the usual flow. It has yet to be demonstrated that this will not affect the distribution within the hepatic arterial bed.

Recent data have demonstrated that the shunt calculated by the use of ^{99m}Tc MAA injection may be significantly higher than the actual shunt of the treatment beads as measured by the posttreatment bremsstrahlung SPECT/CT or positron emission tomography/CT. Since the MAA beads are one-third the diameter of the treatment beads and are more compressible, so they may shunt through smaller connections than the treatment beads, the likelihood of an inaccurate or at least unreliable shunt may be measured. If the

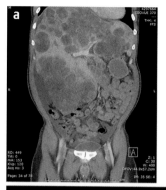

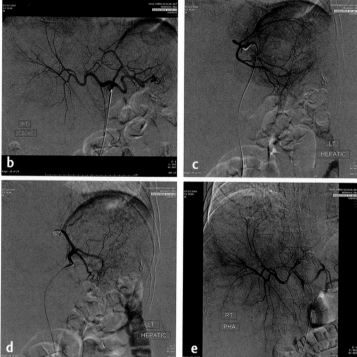

shunt is marginally high, a preliminary bland embolization of the hepatic arteries to be treated has been postulated to decrease the shunt and allow treatment. However, it has been the author's experience that this bland embolization rarely decreases the shunt enough to allow treatment.

If the bilirubin is elevated, an obstructive cause should first be sought to relieve the obstruction via catheter or internal stent drainage. Elevated

Fig. 4.12 A 53-year-old-male with widely metastatic neuroendocrine tumor. He has been treated at an outside hospital with octreotide and Avastin. He wishes to undergo ^{90}Y therapy to palliate his pain. **(a)** Computed tomography demonstrates that the patient has a huge liver with approximately 70% of the volume occupied by tumor. Even with this tumor burden, his bilirubin remains at 1.2 mg/dL. **(b)** The celiac arteriogram shows that the left hepatic artery is replaced to the left gastric artery. This would endanger the stomach if particles were infused so close to the gastric arteries. **(c)** A selective left hepatic arteriogram demonstrates that there is significant tumor vascularity present but no accessory left gastric artery that would supply the stomach fundus. **(d)** The left hepatic artery was embolized with a platinum microcoil so that the intrahepatic collateral vessels would take the yttrium beads to all the liver from a right hepatic arterial embolization. Immediately after the coil was placed, he began complaining of upper abdominal pain. This was, in retrospect, due to the Avastin that prevented tumoral vessels from enlarging and the amount of tumor that was in the left lobe became immediately ischemic since the blood flow was inadequate to fully supply it. **(e)** The right hepatic arteriogram shows the tumor in the right lobe and there is some intrahepatic vessels crossing to the left lobe. The patient was admitted for hydration and pain control overnight and recovered well enough to undergo the yttrium therapy, which did palliate the pain of the expanding tumor.

bilirubin can also be caused by sorafenib. If the patient has been on this drug for several weeks, it is a good idea to temporarily halt the drug for a week or two as the bilirubin may return to normal levels. If the bilirubin does return to more normal levels, the radioembolization may proceed. However, particularly in HCC patients, a bilirubin on the day of treatment should be obtained to ensure that the patient is still a candidate for therapy particularly if the bilirubin level obtained previously was near 2 mg/dL. These patients may deteriorate quickly and, if prior therapy has been performed and radioembolization is a salvage procedure, they need to be followed closely. If the radioembolization procedure is localized to a single segment to eliminate an area of tumor in a segment of the liver, a "radiation segmentectomy," a more aggressive use of radioembolization with delivery of a high dose of beads to an artery serving a single segment sparing the majority of the liver parenchyma, may be an option.

A relative contraindication is the invasion of the portal vein by tumor. While one product (glass beads) views this as a contraindication, there have been reports using the other product (resin beads) to treat these patients and resolve the intraportal tumor so that several patients have had successful liver transplants.[13]

When deciding on the embolic agent, radioembolization, or transarterial chemoembolization (TACE), keep in mind that the TACE particles are larger and will occlude more proximally, making it difficult to treat a tumor distally. The ideal order of therapy is to utilize ^{90}Y beads, which are approximately 40 μ in diameter as many times as is practicable. A time lapse between radioembolization therapies of 3 to 6 months is necessary to allow the normal tissues affected by the radiation to recover, but after that, it may be utilized again. If the patient's bilirubin becomes elevated, it may be necessary to shift to TACE (**Fig. 4.13**).

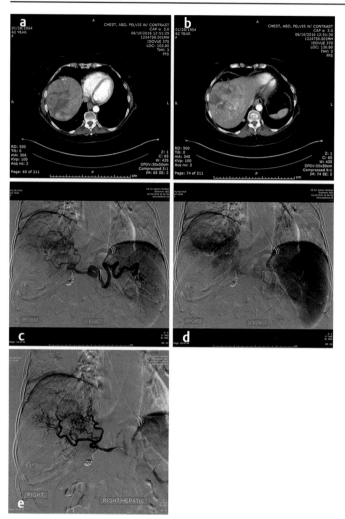

Fig. 4.13 A 62-year-old female presents with recurring hepatocellular carcinoma despite transarterial chemoembolization (TACE) × 3. Now he is being considered for 90Y therapy. **(a,b)** Computed tomography scans demonstrate a large enhancing mass predominantly in the right lobe. **(c)** Celiac axis arteriogram shows the relative lack of vessels in the tumor. **(d)** Late arterial phase demonstrates the mass well in the superior portion of the right lobe. **(e)** Selective right hepatic arteriogram injected at 1 mL/s for a total of 8 mL shows how slow the flow is to the right lobe. This case demonstrates that TACE to begin treatment of hypervascular tumors is incorrect if there is a possibility of using ^{90}Y since the particles used to treat the tumor in TACE are three times larger than those utilized for ^{90}Y. This prevents the smaller particles from lodging in the tumoral vasculature. If tumors recur and the patient cannot tolerate another yttrium treatment, the appropriate treatment is TACE.

Hepatic Arterial Infusion of Chemotherapy

Surgical placement of hepatic arterial pumps has been demonstrated to prolong the progression-free survival of colon cancer patients with liver metastases but not the overall survival. When this therapy is utilized, it is necessary for the surgeon to have the interventional radiologist embolize with coils any aberrant or replaced branches of the hepatic artery so that the entire liver may be perfused with one pump catheter, which is usually placed through the GDA. Coil embolization of such arteries will open, within seconds, the intrahepatic collateral arteries so that the entire liver can be perfused with a single catheter placement. This technique has also been reported to be successful when dealing with a replaced left hepatic artery to the left gastric artery when radioembolization is performed. Coil embolization of the left hepatic artery will open the collaterals to the left lobe eliminating the need to put the gastric arteries at risk by embolizing with the radioactive beads so close to their origins. No difference has been seen where this technique is utilized when compared with radioembolization into the replaced left hepatic artery. It should also be noted that a selective arteriogram of the left hepatic artery should be performed before it is embolized to demonstrate if there is also a connection to the left distal left gastric artery, which could deliver the radioactive particles to the fundus of the stomach or to the gastroesophageal junction. If such a connection is observed, it should be embolized with coils as distally as possible before the left hepatic artery is embolized.

Placement of percutaneous arterial infusion catheters via the subclavian, axillary, or brachial arteries into the liver has been performed so the catheter is then left in place in the liver and infusional chemotherapy is then performed via a port that is placed subcutaneously at the insertion site. The results of this therapy mirror those of the surgically placed pumps for metastatic colon cancer. This technique is predominantly reported in the Japanese and Korean literature.

Percutaneous Biliary Drainage

While endoscopically placed stents have become the standard for biliary drainage, the percutaneous approach cannot be ignored. Originally described in Japanese literature, the approach to the left hepatic ducts was initially preferred because these ducts are closer to the surface than those on the right. However, the radiation dose to the interventional radiologist's hands was greater and subsequently the right ductal approach was developed in the US. If the ducts have been obstructed for days to weeks and are extremely large, it is a relatively straightforward procedure to access them either via the right mid-axillary line or anteriorly into the left lobe with US guidance. US guidance has become the standard to access the ducts as even smaller ones can be accessed, particularly the left ducts. Contrast is injected to determine the anatomy of the ducts and a wire placed into the duct. An angled catheter and a hydrophilic guidewire to place the catheter into the duodenum where a stiffer guidewire is used to support the placement of an internal–external stent then follow. If the wire cannot be passed into the duodenum, a drainage catheter should be placed in the common bile duct to decompress the system externally for 24 to 48 hours to allow any edema from the biliary dilation to resolve and then the internal–external stent placed (**Fig. 4.14**). A temptation is to place an entirely internal stent across the obstruction, but this may lead to tumor ingrowth into the stent obstructing it. Metallic stents should only be placed in patients who have a 6-month life expectancy as that is about the patency period of the metallic stent. Recent endoscopic developments have led to the placement of covered stents from the common bile duct into the left hepatic duct. This isolates the right biliary ducts, which may result in the formation of bilomas and multiple abscesses. Any patient with a covered stent obstructing the ducts of one lobe should be followed closely since the percutaneous placement of a biliary drain can be performed and the drain placed through the covering of the stent to adequately drain the obstructed system (**Fig. 4.15**). Because this can be a long and painful procedure, the use of monitored anesthesia care provided by the anesthesiology department should be considered, as conscious sedation may not be deep enough to adequately sedate the patient.

Angioplasty and Stenting in the Cancer Patient

While peripheral vascular disease (PVD) patients commonly have stenoses and occlusions that require angioplasty and stenting, cancer patients may also suffer from PVD but have some stenoses that are peculiar to the disease process.

Venous stents are utilized in treating the SVC syndrome of upper extremity and facial edema, respiratory difficulty, and headaches, which are due to the tumor compressing the SVC, restricting blood return to the right atrium, and elevating the venous pressure proximal to the stenosis. If possible, these stenoses should be treated before radiation is given to the lung cancer that is compressing the SVC. Since radiation affects small vessels more than large vessels, the vasa vasorum of the SVC are impacted and the stenosis becomes highly fibrotic and difficult to angioplasty and stent. Large, 12 to 18 mm, uncovered balloon expandable or self-expanding

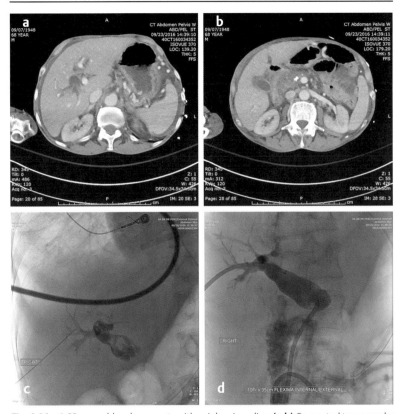

Fig. 4.14   A 68-year-old male presents with painless jaundice. **(a,b)** Computed tomography scans demonstrate enlarged biliary ducts and a mass in the head of the pancreas. **(c)** From a right mid-axillary line, under ultrasound and fluoroscopic guidance, a 21-gauge needle is placed within the dilated right hepatic bile duct. **(d)** The wire went without difficulty into the duodenum and a stent placed across the obstruction. It should be noted that the lead marker on the internal–external stent is where the most proximal side holes are located and should be well within the ductal system.

stents should be used. Placing these patients into a supine position, as the right jugular approach is preferred since it is a straight path to the right atrium, is difficult due to their respiratory status. This initial angioplasty of the stenosis should be performed as quickly as feasible. Patients receive an almost instantaneous response to the relief of pressure allowing the further angioplasty and stenting. If it is impossible for the patient to be completely supine, a brachial or antecubital approach can be utilized (**Fig. 4.16**). A similar procedure can be utilized if the patient has relatively acute onset of lower extremity and abdominal edema due to the encroachment of a tumor mass

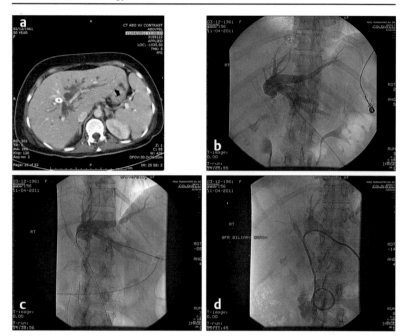

Fig. 4.15   A 50-year-old female with pancreatic carcinoma presents with jaundice and ele-vated bilirubin. Endoscopy performed and covered stent placed in common bile duct directly superiorly into superior right hepatic ducts. **(a)** Computed tomography demonstrates that the stent is occluding the left hepatic duct causing ductal dilatation. **(b)** Percutaneous trans-shepatic cholangiography is performed from a left approach filling the dilated ducts and demonstrating the blockage at the stent. **(c)** A catheter is then placed in the duct and a hydrophilic glidewire is placed through the wall of the covered stent followed by the cathe-ter. **(d)** An internal–external drain is placed through the existing covered stent and into the duodenum, successfully draining the left ducts.

on the inferior vena cava. In fact, the obstruction of the subclavian vein is not uncommon when there are enlarged supraclavicular lymph nodes as seen in melanoma and head and neck cancers. Patients present with cold hands but with demonstrably adequate arterial flow. A stent can then be placed in the subclavian vein to open up the return so that the arterial flow is not compromised (**Fig. 4.17**). The worst cases can result in phlegmasia cerulea dolens.

Arterial stenting is utilized to treat stenoses caused by tumor inva-sion of the artery. Stent grafts are usually used since the graft material will resist the invasion of tumor. This is an uncommon problem but one that can be life-threatening when a head and neck cancer, usually ton-sillar, recurs after radiation and surgery to the original tumor resulting

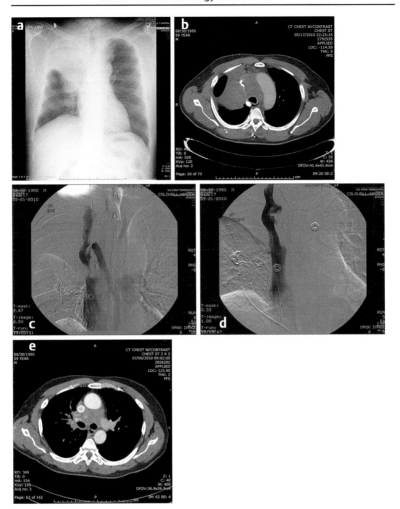

Fig. 4.16 A 59-year-old male presents with shortness of breath, facial swelling, and inability to lie supine with a 50-pack-year history of smoking. **(a)** Posteroanterior chest radiograph demonstrates the collapse of the right upper lobe suggesting a central lesion. **(b)** The computed tomography (CT) scan shows the central non–small cell lung cancer that is obstructing the stromal vascular cell and filling the azygous vein. **(c)** The right internal jugular vein is accessed and a cava-gram obtained showing the high-grade stenosis with filling of the azygous vein. **(d)** A 12-mm diameter self-expanding stent is placed across the lesion relieving the upstream pressure and filled normally into the right atrium. **(e)** A CT performed a month later shows that the stent remains open despite the presence of the lung cancer.

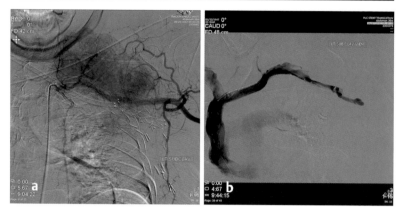

Fig. 4.17 A 56-year-old male with metastatic melanoma to the brachial lymph nodes presents with a chronically cold left hand. **(a)** A subclavian arteriogram demonstrates the size and hypervascularity of the nodes. **(b)** A subclavian venogram demonstrates the stenosis caused by the enlarged nodes restricting venous flow. A 10-mm self-expanding stent was placed at the site of the stenosis restoring venous flow. By the time the patient was taken off the interventional radiology table and into the holding area, his hand was warm.

in a carotid "blowout." This acute rupture of the artery occurs in 2 to 4% of treated head and neck cancers and is fatal in almost all cases, particularly when the patient is not in the hospital (**Fig. 4.18**).

Percutaneous Nephrostomy

Obstruction of the drainage of the kidney is a problem that is often seen in urothelial or gynecologic cancers, where the cancer will grow from either the ureter, bladder, uterus, or cervix and into the ureter/bladder or merely compress these adjacent structures. Obviously sterile technique is observed at all times and the patient placed either prone or prone-decubitus. Adequate sedation and analgesia must be administered to obtain patient compliance and performance of a safe procedure. Versed and fentanyl may be given in the IR area, but there must be a nurse monitoring the patient individually in the IR suite. Under US guidance, the renal collecting system is imaged and a 21-gauge needle inserted into the collecting system followed by a stiff 0.018-inch wire over which a dilator/catheter is placed dilating the tract to 7 Fr. The wire and all the inner components are removed leaving only the 7-Fr sheath in the kidney through which a 0.035-inch wire is placed, followed by several tissue dilators up to the catheter size that is going to be placed in the renal pelvis. The actual puncture should occur in Brody's area,

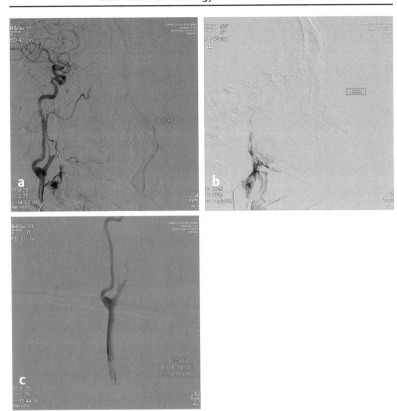

Fig. 4.18 A 48-year-old male with treated squamous cell carcinoma of the tonsil involving surgery and free flap placement, chemotherapy, and radiation presents with massive hemoptysis in the waiting room of the cancer center. A passing physician had the presence of mind to apply direct pressure and bring him directly to the Interventional Radiology suite. **(a)** The lateral view of the common carotid arteriogram demonstrates the contrast leakage near the origin. **(b)** Selective catheterization demonstrates that the contrast is leaking into the posterior pharynx. **(c)** An 8-mm diameter covered stent is placed over the origin of the "blowout," sealing the leak and stabilizing the patient.

which is in the short axis midpoint opposite the renal pelvis. This is the least vascular area in the kidney to minimize the chances of hemorrhage. Placement of a nephrostomy in patients who have had neobladder or "Indiana pouch" surgery with stenosis at the distal anastomotic site and need a stent across the stenosis can have the stent placed in a single session if the stenosis can easily be crossed and the puncture not excessively hemorrhagic. If not, a nephrostomy is placed and the stent placement attempted after 24 to 48 hours of decompression. This time lag allows for the edema around the stenosis to resolve and a channel to open. These patients can have stents placed that are long enough to reach the ileostomy bag so that they can and should be changed on a regular 3-month schedule. Patients with a vesicovaginal fistula, usually a gynecologic malignancy post radiation therapy, are more challenging as the collecting system is not dilated, and to divert the urine flow away from the area, nephrostomies are placed under US guidance. The "two-stick" method is usually used where the pelvis is punctured with a 22-gauge needle, followed by contrast and air injection. The air demonstrates the posterior calyces so that they may be punctured more readily. This technique can also be utilized for any nephrostomy placement.

Pain Management

The alliance of IR and the oncology service allows the use of precision needle placement for oncologic pain management. While this has been an area that has been traditionally the province of the anesthesiologist or pain physician, the placement of blocks by anatomic landmarks without CT or US guidance is both less accurate and less effective. Since the interventional radiologist is an expert at placement of needles under imaging guidance, this is a natural fit and a real service to the management of these patients. Reaching out to the palliative care service and the medical oncologist will allow patients to be referred more readily.

- Nerve blocks are usually placed with an anesthetic and steroid combination to test the effectiveness of the block and to decrease the inflammation due to the tumor compression or involvement. If the block at the level is effective and there are no motor nerves involved, the nerve can be safely ablated with either ethanol or phenol. The nerve blocks that are routinely performed in IR are the following:
  - Intercostal nerve block:
    - Indication: Pain along the chest wall.
    - Procedure: A 22- to 25-gauge needle can be placed approximately 10 cm from the spinous process immediately under the inferior portion of the rib and 5 to 10 mL of ropivacaine/steroid mixture injected initially; then, when proven effective, approximately 5 mL of lidocaine is injected followed by 5 mL of ethanol. If the patient experiences any pain with the ethanol injection, this can be treated with additional lidocaine since the effect is immediate rather than the delay seen when either bupivacaine or ropivacaine is utilized. Care must be taken to avoid the tracking of the ethanol into the spinal canal.

- Celiac plexus block:
  - Indication: Upper abdominal pain due to pancreatic carcinoma, hepatic arterial embolization, large tumors in the liver stretching the liver capsule.
  - Procedure: The patient is placed in the prone position on the CT scanner and the celiac axis identified. The celiac plexus is located immediately superior to the origin of the celiac axis, anterior to the aorta. While the plexus itself is rarely identified, the target for the needle is immediately superior to the celiac axis within a centimeter of the aorta. A route is determined to avoid placement of a needle through the kidney or aorta. A 22-gauge needle is used and either a bilateral or a unilateral approach is used. Once the needle is positioned above the celiac axis, a small amount of dilute contrast is injected to verify position and the distribution of the anesthetic. Either ropivacaine or bupivacaine is used to determine the efficacy of the block. If the block eliminates or significantly reduces the pain, the patient returns for an ablation with 10- to 25-mL ethanol. The same position of the needle may be obtained from an anterior approach, but the bilateral posterior approach, if the plexus lies in the midline, is preferred since there is more uniform and wider distribution of the anesthetic or alcohol (**Fig. 4.19**)
  - Complications: Elimination of the celiac plexus may result in patients having diarrhea or orthostatic hypotension
- Splanchnic block:
  - Indication: Upper to midabdominal pain.
  - Procedure: Similar to the celiac plexus block, but this plexus is immediately superior to the superior mesenteric artery.
- Pudendal block:
  - Indication: Rectal or pelvic pain.
  - Procedure: The pudendal nerve is immediately anterior to ischial spine of the pelvis. It is usually well identified and a bilateral anterior approach to these nerves is preferred. The same local anesthetic solution utilized in the above blocks is again used and only in cases of severe pain from rectal or pelvic tumor, especially, postradiation rectal cancer patients, is the ablation utilized (**Fig. 4.20**).
- Femoral block:
  - Indication: Thigh pain usually from a large tumor mass.
  - Procedure: The femoral artery is located with US and followed to its bifurcation. Just lateral to the bifurcation a hyperechoic small structure will be present, which is the femoral nerve. Because the femoral nerve contains both motor and sensory

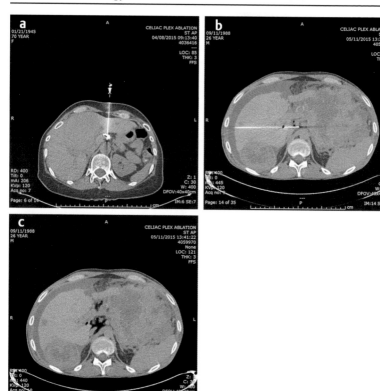

Fig. 4.19 Examples of approaches to place a celiac block/ablation, which should relieve pain in the upper abdomen including liver and pancreas. **(a)** Since the celiac plexus is situated immediately superior to the origin of the celiac axis, a small gauge needle, usually 22 gauge, can be placed into the region from anterior to posterior approach. **(b)** A lateral approach can also be utilized as can a posterior approach. **(c)** The low attenuation area around the celiac plexus is the lidocaine/ethanol mixture.

fibers, if it is anesthetized, the patient may not be able to stand or walk. The patient should be warned about this complication before performance of the block. At the level of the bifurcation, approximately 20 mL of local anesthetic is injected while pressing on the thigh immediately inferior to the puncture site. This will force the anesthetic to move superiorly and anteriorly to effect the more superficial branches and less likely to effect the motor branches.

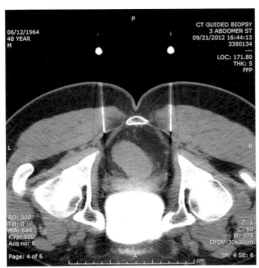

Fig. 4.20 A 46-year-old man presents with unremitting pain due to anal cancer treated with surgery and radiation therapy. Bilateral 20-gauge spinal needles are placed anteriorly to the pudendal nerve where lidocaine followed by ethanol was injected. This immediately resolved his pain and lasted over 6 months. This procedure can be repeated if necessary.

– Stellate ganglion block:
  ▪ Indication: Pain in the face, arm, neck, or chest due to trauma to the sympathetic nerves from surgery or radiation to the area. The anesthesia of this ganglion decreases the norepinephrine that actuates the sympathetic nerves that form the ganglion.
  ▪ Procedure: The stellate ganglion is located immediately laterally to the C6/C7 vertebral body and can be identified on CT of the neck. A 22- to 25-gauge needle is placed from an anterior approach and the ganglion anesthetized. If the anesthesia is properly administered, the patient will have Horner's syndrome with drooping of the eyelid, hoarseness of the voice, and redness of the eye after the procedure. These symptoms will disappear after a few hours to a day.
– Facial nerve block:
  ▪ Indication: Facial nerve pain originating from a tumor involving any branch of the facial nerve. Since the facial nerve is made up of three distinct branches, ophthalmic (serving the forehead), maxillary (serving the midface), and mandibular (serving the lower face and mandible), it is necessary to identify the cause of the pain and in which distribution it lies.
  ▪ Procedure: The injection site is tailored to fit the symptoms. If the mandibular branch of the facial nerve is responsible for the pain, it is easily accessible at the angle of the mandible on the medial side. If it is the ophthalmic branch, it is accessed near

the parotid gland. The maxillary branch is also accessed where it exits the parotid. The entire facial nerve may be treated, but facial droop is expected and the patient should be warned.

- Occipital block:
  - Indication: Metastatic or primary tumor on the posteroinferior aspect of the skull.
  - Procedure: The occipital nerve may be located with US in the neck after it arises from C1/C2 or posterior to the ear. The area is then injected with anesthetic.
- Epidural block:
  - Indication: Chronic back pain that cannot be controlled with oral medications.
  - Procedure: A paramedian approach is utilized at the level of L3 or L4 with the patient prone. A 20- to 22-gauge needle is advanced until the ligamentum flavum is encountered. A syringe with saline or air is attached to the needle after the release of resistance is noted. The saline is preferable to air since the headache is less severe after the procedure. When the epidural space is reached, a combination of steroids and anesthetic is placed. Insure that the dura mater, the covering of the spinal cord, is not punctured by the needle through the use of either fluoroscopy or US.
  - An alternative procedure to place steroids and an anesthetic in place is to place the small needle through a paramedian approach with the tip immediately superficial to the exiting nerve root at a particular interspace where the greatest pain is located. The medications are then injected from 1 to 2 mm away from the nerve and they will track back into the epidural space. This is best performed under CT guidance.
- Back Pain due to Bony Metastatic Disease

  - Indication: Severe pain that is unremitting due to metastases to the vertebrae. A displacement of a bone fragment more than 2 mm into the spinal canal is a contraindication to intervention as the procedure may cause the fragment to track further into the canal and cause a neural deficit.
  - Procedure: There are numerous manufacturers of vertebral augmentation equipment. All have in common that the initial bone biopsy needle is placed either through the pedicle and into the vertebral body or from a parapedicular approach near the pedicle but entering the vertebral body from the lateral cortex of the vertebral body. Once the major access needle is inside the vertebral body, tools may be placed through the needle to create channels, utilize balloon tamps, or RFA probes or cement

delivered directly. The newer types of vertebral augmentation devices supply thicker polymethyl methacrylate cement that can be more easily controlled, reducing the incidence of any cement tracking posteriorly into the spinal canal. Since the vertebral body is involved with tumor, ablation of the tumor should be performed with an RFA probe although cryotherapy has been utilized. This allows the formation of a cavity and eliminating tumor cells. Cement is then delivered until the cement crosses the midline from a unipedicular approach or meets in the center from a bipedicular approach. The cement is then placed within the vertebral body until the upper and lower cortices are resisting the flow of the cement. However, with many tumors, the cortices are not intact and there may be leakage of the cement into the superior or inferior disk spaces or the soft tissues anteriorly or laterally. None of these leakages are particularly dangerous except that anteriorly the cement may enter the Batson's plexus. Careful observation with fluoroscopy or CT will prevent this from occurring. If the posterior wall of the vertebral body is not intact, there is the potential of leakage of cement into the spinal canal. If that should occur, an increase in pain resulting in emergent surgery may be required. Again, familiarity with the properties of the cement with which one is working is necessary for the performance of a safe and effective procedure. With the newer tools available, a unipedicular approach is more common since the risk of perforating the pedicle with the bone biopsy needle is halved and the cement can be provided with a low resistance track to follow (**Fig. 4.21**).

– Results: In patients with multiple types of malignancies metastatic to the spine, patients can expect their pain level to decrease significantly, often from 8 to 10/10 on the visual assessment pain scale to a 0 to 1/10. This has significantly decreased the amounts of medications these patients consume and improved their quality of life.

• Bony Metastatic Disease

– Indications: A bony metastasis that is causing the patient pain whether it has been irradiated or not. The "knee-jerk" response of many physicians taking care of patients with bony metastases is to refer them for external beam radiation. This method of therapy has a 60 to 70% success rate and usually takes about 6 weeks to take effect. Often, there is a single metastasis that may be treated with local measures by RFA and instillation of PMMA cement. This single lesion may allow the patient to undergo his full

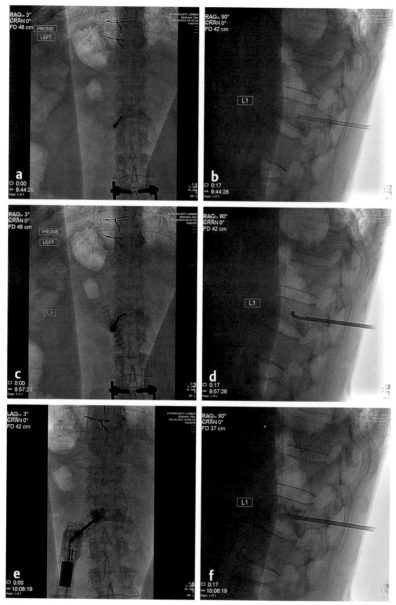

Fig. 4.21 A 75-year-old male with multiple myeloma fell and had a vertebral body compression fracture of L1 and a pain level of 9/10. Previous studies had implicated a tumor at

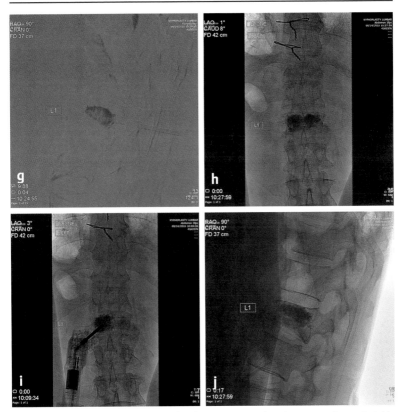

Fig. 4.21 *(Continued)* the L1 level. **(a,b)** The patient was placed prone on the angio table under general anesthesia and a 10-gauge bone trocar placed through the left pedicle into the vertebral body. Biplane fluoroscopy was utilized and is invaluable for these procedures. Procedures on the upper thoracic/cervical spine and the pelvis utilize computed tomography. **(c,d)** A bipolar radiofrequency ablation probe was utilized to treat the tumor tissue within the vertebral body after a bone biopsy had been performed. The radiofrequency ablation probe was also able to cut a channel through the vertebral body through which thick polymethyl methacrylate cement was to flow. It was intended that only a unipedicular approach would be used. **(e,f,g)** The cement is seen flowing into the left side only. The margins of the cement are "fluffy" due to the intercalation of the cement between the trabeculae of the vertebral body. Unfortunately, the cement did not cross the midline so another trocar was placed into the right pedicle. **(h)** When the cement was to start being delivered, a roadmap image of the current cement distribution was obtained and the new cement can be seen filling the right side of the vertebral body. **(i,j)** At the end of the procedure, good cement delivery can be seen both in the anteroposterior and lateral projections. The patient awakened from anesthesia, and noted before going home, that his pain level was 0.

treatment of radiation or leave that until later if only a handful of lesions are present.

- Procedure: This is very similar to the vertebral augmentation described earlier, but other areas are targeted such as the pelvis, femur, or humerus. The targeted bone is entered with the bone biopsy needle, an RFA is performed, and the tumor reinforced with the cement. In larger areas such as the pelvis, additional cement is usually necessary to fill the bone defects. Careful planning of the treatment is required so that each of the defects can be treated and filled maximally. If either the cement or the RFA probe comes into contact with large nerves, the patient may have nerve damage and a walking or gait deficit. It is vitally important to consider the route of the nerves as they exit through the sacral foramina or in the pelvis so that there is no injury. These procedures are usually performed under general anesthesia (**Fig. 4.22**).

• Abdominal Pain due to Mass Effect

It is a common occurrence to have a patient present with significant abdominal pain due to an enlarging mass. While this mass may be a primary tumor, it is most likely due to liver metastases. As the liver enlarges, the capsule around it stretches and, since it is well enervated, causes excruciating pain. A celiac plexus or mesenteric plexus block/ablation may help, but the sheer size of the mass impinging on other organs and parasitizing blood flood flow may render this therapy less effective. Bland (particles only) or chemoembolization may help in shrinking the mass and softening it immediately. For this palliative procedure, there is little justification for chemotherapy added to the mixture since the aim is for immediate tumor response. If the tumor may be separated from the normal vasculature, the smallest available particles may be utilized (40 µ) to begin and then slowly work up to the 100-µ particles (**Fig. 4.23**). This will form a solid barrier to blood flow and cause the tumor to start necrosing immediately. This in turn may yield tumor lysis syndrome if the tumor is large enough to flood the renal tubules causing renal damage. Pretreatment with allopurinol is a good idea when a large tumor mass is embolized. Postembolization syndrome (PES) is also likely to occur. This is a combination of severe pain, nausea, vomiting, and, if in the liver, a rapid increase in liver enzymes. This should be expected after any hepatic or renal embolization where the arterial blood supply is completely obstructed. This is managed as an inpatient since a patient-controlled anesthetic is utilized, usually morphine or dilaudid. This syndrome is not amenable to outpatient management since dehydration and significant pain may often result.

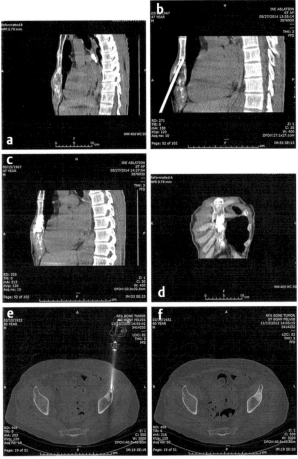

Fig. 4.22 A 47-year-old male with metastatic colon cancer to his sternum causing him excruciating pain. **(a)** The sagittal reconstruction of the computed tomography of the chest demonstrates that the sternum is enlarged where the metastasis is located. **(b)** The bone access needle is placed within the tumor and it ablated with radiofrequency ablation and filled with polymethyl methacrylate (PMMA) cement. **(c,d)** The sagittal and coronal reconstructions from the computed tomography (CT) scan demonstrate that there is excellent filling of the tumor with cement. Upon awakening from general anesthesia, the patient had no pain and this continued until his demise a year later. An 80-year-old male with sclerotic prostate cancer metastasis to his left hip. **(e)** This CT demonstrates the placement of the bipolar radiofrequency ablation probe within the tumor. The tumor was sclerotic enough so that a bone drill had to be used to place the probe. The probe heated the tumor to 60°C and was then removed. The metastasis was too dense to allow any PMMA cement to be utilized. **(f)** This CT shows the tract of the probe through the tumor. This was completely effective and the patient had no pain upon waking up from general anesthesia. He played golf 2 days later.

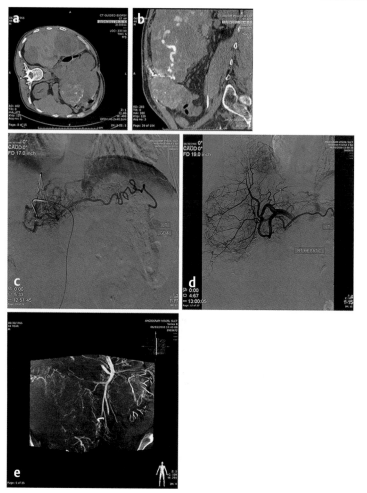

Fig. 4.23 A 46-year-old male presents with a 14-year history of a slowly growing inoperable hemangiopericytoma that originated in his omentum. This tumor produced an insulinlike substance that drove him to originally present in hypoglycemic shock. He had prior chemotherapy to no effect. Now he presents with liver metastases. **(a)** The axial computed tomography demonstrates the large mass filling the patient's abdomen. **(b)** The sagittal reconstruction gives a better idea of how much of the abdomen is filled with tumor. **(c)** The right hepatic arteriogram shows the hypervascular metastases in his liver. **(d)** During the workup for ^{90}Y therapy, the gastroduodenal artery was studied and the visualized gastroepiploic artery demonstrates the connection to a fast filling epiploic artery that supplied the majority of the tumor. **(e)** A cone beam arteriogram demonstrates, on injection of the superior mesenteric artery, that tumor vascularity has parasitized much of the circulation. After multiple embolotherapy treatments, his use of intravenous glucose to combat the hypoglycemic shock was unnecessary and lived for almost 3 years after these treatments began.

Other sources of abdominal pain that are responsive to intra-arterial therapy include the following:

- Recurrent head and neck tumors in the previously maximally irradiated tumor bed. The temptation in many institutions is to re-irradiate even though the patient has received 90 to 100 Gy that will likely lead to necrosis of the area even including the carotid and its branches. Rather than risk this possibility, an intra-arterial infusion of Cisplatin (Platinol) at a modest dose of 30 to 50 mg/m2 can be performed into the artery feeding the original tumor if a branch of the external carotid artery. Caution must be taken not to allow any reflux of the infusate into the internal carotid artery since it can be toxic to the ophthalmic nerve causing blindness. If a standard microcatheter that utilizes a 0.014-inch wire is used to superselectively catheterize the tumor arterial branch, the chemotherapy can be delivered either by using a Harvard-style syringe pump or by merely delivering by manual compression on a 50-mL syringe. The usual dose will take 20 to 30 minutes to infuse by either method. This can be repeated every other week until the pain is relieved. The tumors are also usually sensitive to this chemotherapy, and may actually shrink. The neurotoxic effects of Platinol are used to injure the pain nerves in the distribution of the tumor and pain is relieved in approximately 70% of patients. Additionally, Platinol causes a "radiation recall effect." This effect mimics the effects of dose of an external beam radiation: the tissues inflamed with the actual radiation port may be seen outlined on the patient's skin. The tumor cells react as though they were just radiated. The mechanism of action of this effect is not known (**Fig. 4.24**).
- Postradiation rectal and gynecologic cancer patients. These patients have also been irradiated to their maximum dose and often breakthrough pain that is unmanageable occurs. The same regimen as above may be utilized to treat the pain of these patients also. Bleeding may also occur from pseudoaneurysms formed or from the breakdown of tissues (**Fig. 4.25**).
- Osteosarcoma in the appendicular skeleton. Large osteosarcomas are extremely painful for the patient and a bridge to surgery may be the utilization of intra-arterial infusion of Platinol. This may be a one-time treatment but multiple may be necessary dependent on the ability to get the patient to an accomplished orthopaedic oncologist.
- Large hypervascular tumors not arising in the liver. If their vasculature can be isolated from normal tissues, any embolic agent may be utilized. The radioembolization agents may even be used if there are liver metastases present to justify their

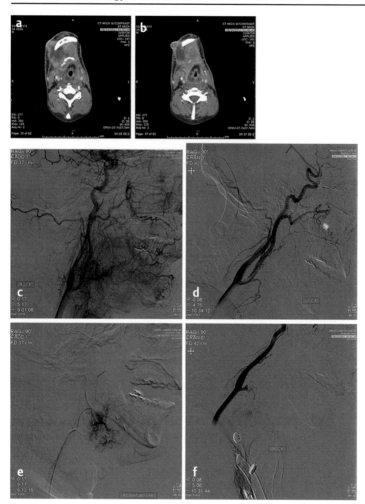

Fig. 4.24 A 36-year-old male with a history of previously treated squamous cell carcinoma of the base of tongue. He had received maximum radiation therapy of 100 Gy and progressed both locally and into lymph nodes. He was in unremitting 10/10 pain that was not able to be effectively treated with routine pain medications. **(a,b)** Computed tomography (CT) scans demonstrating the extensive nature of the recurrence. **(c)** Right common carotid arteriogram demonstrating the hypervascular mass seen on the CT scan which is supplied by the external carotid branches. **(d)** Left common carotid arteriogram showing that there is little supply to the tumor from the opposite side. **(e)** Arteriogram of the right superior thyroidal artery that demonstrates the hypervascular nodal recurrence. This artery and the facial artery were both infused with a dose of 50 mg/m2 of cisplatin dividing the dose equally between the arteries. **(f)** After two treatments to each artery, the right common carotid artery demonstrates that the external carotid artery is no longer patent.

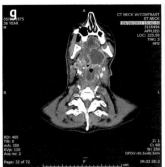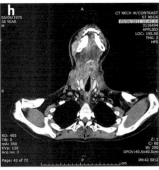

Fig. 4.24 *(Continued)* **(g,h)** The CT scan of the neck demonstrates the necrotic primary tumor as well as the necrotic lymph nodes. More importantly, the patient no longer complained of any pain. This was effective until his demise about 3 months later.

use. Bland embolization will shrink the tumor and decrease any endocrine function, but there may be transient pain (**Fig. 4.26**; **Fig. 4.27**).
• Hemorrhage due to Tumor Invasion of Adjacent Structures

Such invasion is common in high-grade aggressive malignancies. The major problem is deciding what tissues may be sacrificed or put at risk to treat the underlying malignancy. Obviously a hollow viscus should not be embolized with small particles, and postsurgical patients who have had their upper abdominal anatomy altered or removed are at greater risk of postembolization complications since the collateral vessels have been either tied off or removed. Attention to both the size of particle and the ability to keep the embolics away from normal tissues will affect the success of the procedure. However, if there are tissues that may be sacrificed, for example, splenic, hepatic, or renal, the consequences are not as dire as that of a hollow viscus. These organs usually scar down without abscess formation. Palliation of both pain and hemoptysis may be obtained by embolizing the bronchial arteries. Caution must be used to avoid the embolization of the anterior spinal artery via branches of the intercostal bronchial trunk or via neovascularity formed after radiation of a tumor. Embolization of the anterior spinal artery may result in paraplegia that may be temporary or permanent. In no circumstance should liquid embolics or chemotherapy be added to the embolic mixture due to the risk of anterior spinal arterial embolization (**Fig. 4.28**).

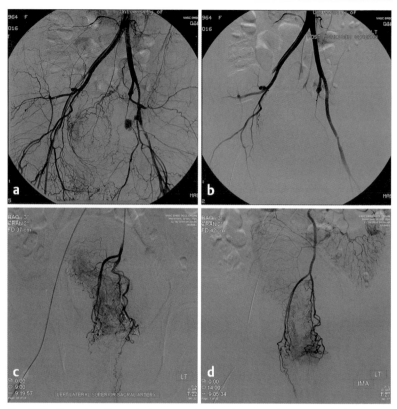

Fig. 4.25 Examples of standard interventional radiology techniques applied to tumor patients. **(a)** A 48-year-old female with a history of fallopian tube cancer and is now stasis post-surgery and radiation therapy. She is noted to have brief episodes of pelvic hemorrhage. The arteriogram demonstrates the pseudoaneurysm of the left external iliac artery. **(b)** A covered stent was placed, which solved the problem. **(c,d)** A 55-year-old male with history of rectal cancer having had a resection and radiation therapy. He presents with arterial bleeding per rectum. An arteriogram shows the pseudoaneurysms likely caused by the radiation therapy. These were then embolized, stopping the bleeding.

Preoperative Embolization

When renal tumors, in particular, are to be surgically removed either via open or laparoscopic approaches, the tumor itself may be embolized with bland particles to minimize blood loss. Ethanol has also been used to sclerose the kidney, but coils should be utilized to occlude the main renal artery so that no re-canalization can occur. If embolizing the right kidney,

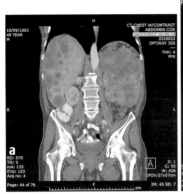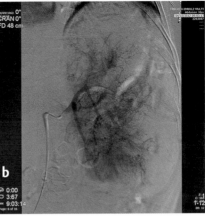

Fig. 4.26 A 48-year-old male presents with left-flank pain that has been growing in intensity for 6 months and now has gross hematuria. **(a)** Computed tomography coronal reconstruction demonstrates the large left upper quadrant mass and liver metastases. The liver metastases were biopsied and shown to be sarcomatoid renal cell carcinoma. **(b)** A renal arteriogram shows the lack of any recognizable renal tissue among all the tumor vascularity. The artery was embolized to stasis and the hematuria stopped.

remember that the right renal artery passes either anteriorly or posteriorly around the IVC so placement of the coils should allow the urologist enough length of artery to place the surgical tie. Preoperative embolization should be performed no more than 24 hours prior to the surgery so that any collateral vessel formation is not a problem. Numerous studies have shown that operative blood loss is significantly lower when preoperative embolization is utilized. This technique may also be used in the orthopaedic management of bone primary or metastatic tumors to reduce blood loss.

Paracentesis and Thoracentesis

Oncology patients often present with benign or malignant effusions or ascites. Both are managed in similar ways. The largest pocket of the fluid collection is localized with US and the skin marked, prepped, and anesthetized with lidocaine with a 25-gauge needle until fluid can be withdrawn or the loss of pressure felt as the needle passes from soft tissue into fluid. A 5-Fr catheter on a needle is then placed through the anesthetized site into the fluid and as much ascites as possible is removed but only 1 to 1.5 L of pleural effusion. Withdrawal of more than this amount of effusion does not assist in the re-inflation of the lung but exacerbates electrolyte shifts. If the fluid re-accumulates, a

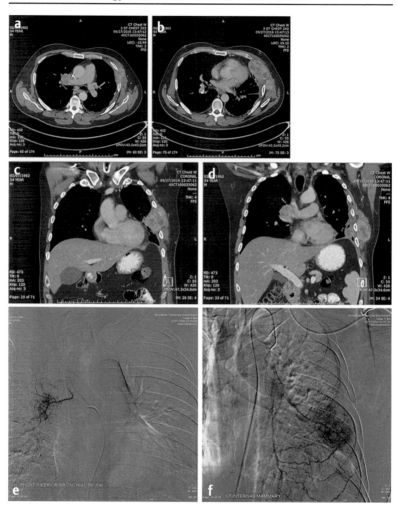

Fig. 4.27 A 54-year-old male with a history of metastatic renal cell carcinoma presents with hemoptysis and severe chest wall pain due to a large mass. **(a)** Axial computed tomography (CT) demonstrates the large chest wall mass that enhances with contrast. **(b)** Axial CT shows the metastatic node in the right hilum. **(c)** Coronal reconstruction gives a better idea of the extent of the chest wall mass. **(d)** Coronal reconstruction demonstrates the metastatic node in the right hilum. **(e)** Bronchial arteriogram shows the hypervascular nature of the tumor. This was embolized to stasis with 100-μ-diameter particles. The patient did not complain of hemoptysis after this procedure. **(f)** Left internal mammary arteriogram demonstrates the hypervascular chest wall mass fed from the left anterior fifth and sixth intercostal arteries. Both of these arteries were embolized to stasis with 100-μ-diameter particles.

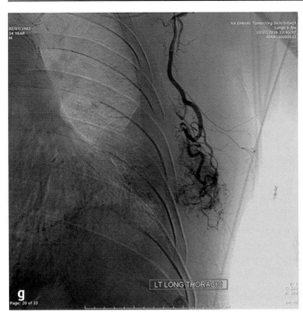

Fig. 4.27 *(Continued)* **(g)** The long thoracic artery arteriogram shows that this artery is very enlarged and is the major supply to the chest wall mass. Again, this was embolized to stasis with 100-μ-diameter particles. The patient initially complained of severe pain at the site of his chest wall mass, but that subsided and after a few days was nontender and well palliated.

more permanent catheter may be placed. Such a catheter is placed via an US localization of the fluid and a guidewire placed into the fluid using an 18-gauge needle in the usually prepped, draped, and anesthetized region. A 10-cm tunnel is then anesthetized and the stab entry site is made on the skin staying clear of places where the belt or undergarments may irritate the catheter site. This 16-Fr catheter is tunneled from the skin site to the entry site and placed into the chronic fluid collection. The catheter has a valve so that no air is insufflated. Vacuum bottles are given to the patient and the patient may drain their fluid at home without having to return to the hospital. Since the ascites may require multiple bottles, a field expedient of using the plastic 16-gauge intravenous line (without the needle) is attached to an extension line and placed through the diaphragm and the free end into a urinal placed on the floor next to the patient. This allows the drainage to proceed and the patient may measure their output. These chronic catheters are usually placed after serial thoracenteses/paracenteses to determine the frequency of the drainage. Once the drainage intervals are less than a month apart, chronic catheters are an option.

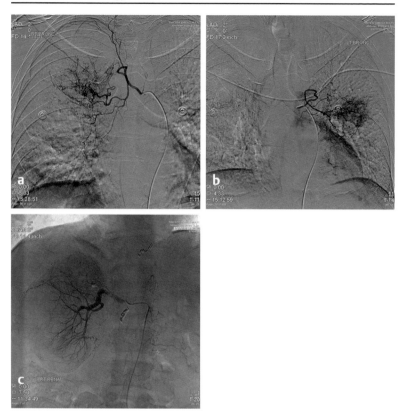

Fig. 4.28 A 64-year-old male with transitional cell carcinoma (TCC) of the right kidney presents with hemoptysis due to pulmonary metastases and hematuria. **(a,b)** Bilateral bronchial arteriograms demonstrating the hypervascularity due to the metastases to the hila. These were both embolized with immediate cessation of the bleeding. The patient made the observation a few weeks later that he was coughing up pieces of necrotic tumor but found this far preferable to blood. **(c)** The right renal arteriogram shows the avascular area in the inferior half of the kidney that represents the TCC. This inferior half was embolized with particles and his hematuria stopped.

References

1. Shi F, Tan Z, An H, Wang X, Xu Y, Wang S. Hepatocellular carcinoma ≤ 4 cm treated with radiofrequency ablation with or without percutaneous ethanol injection. Ann Hepatol 2016;15(1):61–70

2 Georgiades CS, Rodriguez R. Efficacy and safety of percutaneous cryoablation for stage 1A/B renal cell carcinoma: results of a prospective, single-arm, 5-year study. Cardiovasc Intervent Radiol 2014;37(6):1494–1499

3 Breen DJ, Bryant TJ, Abbas A, et al. Percutaneous cryoablation of renal tumours: outcomes from 171 tumours in 147 patients. BJU Int 2013;112(6):758–765

4 Bhonsle S, Bonakdar M, Neal RE II, et al. Characterization of irreversible electroporation ablation with a validated perfused organ model. J Vasc Interv Radiol 2016;27(12):1913–1922.e2

5 Martin RC II, McFarland K, Ellis S, Velanovich V. Irreversible electroporation in locally advanced pancreatic cancer: potential improved overall survival. Ann Surg Oncol 2013;20(Suppl 3):S443–S449

6 Schulz B, Ou J, Van Meter T, Martin RC. Early nontumorous CT findings after irreversible electroporation of locally advanced pancreatic cancer. Abdom Radiol (NY) 2016;41(11):2142–2149

7 Samman M, Mujo T, Harris JJ, Coldwell DM, Hite–Potts M, Vyleta M. Subcutaneous Port Malfunction: A retrospective comparison between internal jugular and subclavian vein access. J Assoc Vasc Access 2015;20(4):229–234

8 Harris J, Mujo T, Potts M, Coldwell D. When is port salvage a feasible option? J Vasc Interv Radiol 2016;27(3):S89

9 Kruskal JB, Hlatky L, Hahnfeldt P, Teramoto K, Stokes KR, Clouse ME. In vivo and in vitro analysis of the effectiveness of doxorubicin combined with temporary arterial occlusion in liver tumors. J Vasc Interv Radiol 1993;4(6):741–747

10 Brown KT, Do RK, Gonen M, et al. Randomized trial of hepatic artery embolization for hepatocellular carcinoma using doxorubicin-eluting microspheres compared with embolization with microspheres alone. J Clin Oncol 2016;34(17):2046–2053

11 Irie K, Morimoto M, Numata K, et al. Enhancement of radiofrequency ablation of the liver combined with transarterial embolization using various embolic agents. Abdom Imaging 2015;40(6):1821–1828

12 Sangro B, Gil-Alzugaray B, Rodriguez J, et al. Liver disease induced by radioembolization of liver tumors: description and possible risk factors. Cancer 2008;112(7):1538–1546

13 Ettorre GM, Levi Sandri GB, Laurenzi A, et al. Yttrium-90 radioembolization for hepatocellular carcinoma prior to liver transplantation. World J Surg Surg 2017;41(1):241–249

5 Chemotherapeutic Agents

Douglas M. Coldwell

Abraxane, see Paclitaxel
Adriamycin, see Doxorubicin
Allopurinol

Type: Antihyperuricemic agent.
Method of action: Xanthine oxidase inhibitor.
Half-life: 2 hours.
Metabolized: Liver.
Excretion: Feces.
Indications: Originally gout but hyperuricemia as part of tumor lysis
  syndrome, which occurs when large volumes of tumors become
  necrotic and can obstruct the renal tubules. When large tumors are
  embolized, oral allopurinol therapy can be started several days in
  advance at 300 mg every 12 hours.
Side effects:
  • Unusual: Skin rash, fever, eosinophilia, hepatitis, decreased renal
    function, Stevens–Johnson syndrome.

Amifostine

Type: Organic hypophosphate prodrug that is hydrolyzed to the active
  cytoprotective drug.
Method of action: Free radical scavenger within cells.
Half-life: 8 minutes.
Metabolized: Liver.
Excretion: Feces.
Indications: Cytoprotective agent to reduce renal toxicity from cisplatin
  and neutropenia-induced fever.
Side effects:
  • Common: diarrhea, hypocalcemia, nausea, vomiting.
  • Serious: Hypotension (in over 60%), cutaneous rash, Stevens–
    Johnson syndrome, toxic epidermal necrolysis, rash.

BCNU (Carmustine)

Type: Nitrogen mustard alkylating agent.
Method of action: Forms links between deoxyribonucleic acid (DNA) strands preventing replication and transcription.
Half-life: 1.4 minutes.
Metabolized: Liver.
Excretion: Urine.
Indications: Brain tumors as it will cross the blood–brain barrier, multiple myeloma, Hodgkin's disease, Non-Hodgkin's lymphoma.
Side effects: Seizures, hemiplegia, headache, metabolic disorder, somnolence, fever.

Bevacizumab (Avastin)

Type: Angiogenesis inhibitor.
Method of action: Monoclonal antibody binding to vascular endothelial growth factor-A inhibiting the formation of tumor neovascularity.
Half-life: 20 days.
Excretion: Systemic.
Indications: Colon, lung, renal, ovarian cancers, glioblastoma multiforme.
Side effects: Inhibition of wound healing, arterial dissection, bleeding, bowel perforation, fatigue, infection, thrombotic microangiopathy, necrotizing fasciitis.

Bleomycin

Type: Byproduct of bacterium *Streptomyces verticillus.*
Method of action: Induces DNA strand breaks and may inhibit the incorporation of thymidine into DNA.
Half-life: 2 hours.
Metabolized: Liver.
Excretion: Urine.
Indications: Hodgkin's/non-Hodgkin's disease, testicular, ovarian cervical cancers.
Side effects: Pulmonary fibrosis with oxygen sensitivity, fever, alopecia, Raynaud's phenomenon (secondary Raynaud's).

Capecitabine (Xeloda)

Type: Oral prodrug that forms 5-fluorouracil (5FU) by thymidine phosphorylase in tumor tissue.

Method of action: Inhibits DNA synthesis during S phase by thymidylate synthetase inhibition.

Half-life: 0.75 hours.

Metabolized: Liver.

Excretion: Urine.

Indications: Colon cancer, breast cancer.

Side effects: Increases effects of warfarin and increases INR (international normalized ratio). Nausea, diarrhea, cardiotoxicity, hand–foot syndrome, severe mucocutaneous reactions such as Stevens–Johnson syndrome and toxic epidermal necrolysis.

Carmustine, see BCNU

Cetuximab (Erbitux)

Type: Monoclonal antibody to human epidermal growth factor receptor (EGFR).

Method of action: Prevents uncontrolled growth via the EGF pathway but must have KRAS (V-Ki-ras2 Kirsten rat sarcoma viral oncogene homolog) wild-type receptor.

Half-life: 114 hours.

Excretion: Systemic.

Indications: KRAS wild-type colorectal carcinoma, head and neck cancer, non–small cell lung cancer.

Side effects: Dermatologic reaction, erythema, acneiform dermatitis, pruritus, hypomagnesemia, fatigue, abdominal pain, nausea, diarrhea/constipation, vomiting.

Rare: pulmonary or cardiac toxicity.

Cyclophosphamide (Cytoxan)

Type: Alkylating antineoplastic.

Method of Action: Cross-linking with tumor DNA, not cell cycle stage specific, immunosuppressive.

Half-life: 3 to 12 hours.

Metabolized: Liver.

Excretion: Feces.

Indications: Non-Hodgkin's lymphoma (NHL), breast cancer.

Side Effects: Immunosuppression, hemorrhagic cystitis, radiation recall effect.

Dacarbazine (DTIC)

Type: Alkylating agent for both DNA and ribonucleic acid (RNA).
Method of Action: Causes DNA double-strand breaks and apoptosis.
Half-life: 5 hours.
Metabolized: Liver.
Excretion: Urine.
Indications: Hodgkin's disease, metastatic melanoma.
Side effects: Nausea, vomiting, leukopenia, thrombocytopenia, hypersensitivity.

Daunorubicin

Type: Anthracycline antitumor antibiotic.
Method of Action: Intercalates between DNA base pairs and inhibits topoisomerase II.
Half-life: 18.5 to 26 hours.
Metabolized: Liver.
Excretion: Feces.
Indications: Acute nonlymphocytic leukemia, acute lymphocytic leukemia.
Side Effects: Nausea, vomiting, cardiac arrhythmias.

Docetaxel (Taxotere)

Type: Semisynthetic taxane.
Method of Action: Prevents depolymerization of cellular microtubules resulting in DNA, RNA, and protein synthesis inhibition.
Half-life: 11 hours.
Metabolized: Liver.
Excretion: Urine.
Indications: Breast cancer, non–small cell lung cancer, gastric cancer, head and neck cancer, prostate cancer (with prednisone).
Side effects: Peripheral neuropathy, stomatitis, renal or hepatic impairment, neutropenia, diarrhea, thrombocytopenia, alopecia.

Doxorubicin (Adriamycin)

Type: Anthracycline antitumor antibiotic.
Method of action: Intercalates with tumor DNA preventing the action of the enzyme topoisomerase II cleaving the DNA and results in apoptosis.
Half-life: 1 to 3 hours.
Metabolized: Liver.
Excretion: Urine, feces.
Indications: Bladder, breast, stomach, lung, ovaries, thyroid, soft-tissue sarcoma, multiple myeloma.
Side Effects: Cardiac toxicity, myelosuppression, alopecia.

Epirubicin

Type: Anthracycline antitumor antibiotic.
Method of action: Intercalates with tumor DNA preventing the action of the enzyme topoisomerase II cleaving the DNA and results in apoptosis.
Half-life: 31 to 35 hours.
Metabolized: Liver.
Excretion: Feces.
Indications: Breast cancer.
Side effects: Hepatic and renal dysfunction, bone marrow dysfunction, neutropenia, alopecia, nausea, vomiting, leukopenia, thrombocytopenia, amenorrhea, anemia, mucositis.

Epoetin Alfa (EPO, Procrit, Epogen)

Type: Hematopoietic growth factor.
Method of action: Stimulates erythropoiesis via division and differentiation in bone marrow.
Half-life: 16 to 67 hours.
Metabolized: Liver.
Excretion: Feces.
Indications: Anemia due to chemotherapy or kidney disease, preparation for surgery with high risk of blood loss.
Side Effects: Fever, nausea, hypertension, cough, vomiting, pruritus, rash, headache, arthralgias.

Erbitux, see Cetuximab
Erlotinib (Tarceva)

Type: Small molecule tyrosine kinase inhibitor.
Method of action: Binds to EGFR and inhibits the production of tyrosine kinase.
Half-life: 36.2 hours.
Metabolized: Liver.
Excretion: Feces.
Indications: Non–small cell lung cancer, locally advanced pancreatic cancer.
Side effects: Acneiform rash (which is thought to be a marker of clinical benefit), erythema, pruritus, fatigue, diarrhea.

Etoposide (VP-16)

Type: Topoisomerase inhibitor.
Method of action: Inhibits DNA replication with G2-phase arrest and preferentially killing cells in G2 or late S phase.
Half-life: 6 to 12 hours.
Metabolized: Liver.
Excretion: Urine.
Indications: Testicular cancer, small cell lung cancer, Kaposi's sarcoma, Ewing's sarcoma, lymphoma, glioblastoma multiforme.
Side effects: Severe myelosuppression with bleeding and infection, leukopenia, thrombocytopenia, nausea, vomiting, alopecia, anorexia, diarrhea, anemia.

Filgrastim (GCSF, Neupogen)

Type: Granulocyte colony–stimulating factor.
Method of action: Recombinant DNA origin to stimulate the proliferation and differentiation of granulocytes.
Half-life: 1.8 to 3.5 hours.
Excretion: Degraded systemically.
Indications: Neutropenia.
Side effects: Nausea, vomiting, bone pain, alopecia, diarrhea, fever, fatigue, hypersensitivity, hypersplenism with rupture (rare), alveolar hemorrhage, hemoptysis.

5-Fluorouracil (5-FU)

Type: Antimetabolite and pyrimidine analog.
Method of Action: Irreversible inhibition of thymidylate synthetase.
Half-life: 16 minutes.
Metabolized: Liver.
Excretion: Urine.
Indications: Anal, breast, colorectal, esophageal, stomach, pancreatic cancers.
Side effects: Mucositis, hand–foot syndrome, cardiac toxicity, myelosuppression.
Related drugs: Capecitabine (oral and converted to 5-FU in tumor).

Floxuridine (FUDR)

Type: Antimetabolite.
Method of action: Metabolized to an active metabolite of 5-FU that inhibits thymidylate synthetase.
Half-life: 16 minutes.
Metabolized: Liver.
Excretion: Urine.
Indications: Gastrointestinal adenocarcinoma.
Side effects: Nausea, vomiting, diarrhea, mucositis, myelosuppression, anemia.

Folinic Acid, see Leucovorin
Gemcitabine (Gemzar)

Type: Pyrimidine analog.
Method of action: Kills cells in S phase while undergoing DNA synthesis.
Half-life: 42 to 94 minutes for short infusions.
Metabolized: Liver.
Excretion: Urine.
Indications: Pancreatic cancer, non–small cell lung cancer, breast cancer, ovarian cancer, bladder cancer, cholangiocarcinoma.
Side effects: Nausea, vomiting, anemia, hepatic dysfunction, myelosuppression, pain, fever, hematuria, dyspnea, rash, hemorrhage, infection, alopecia, radiation recall effect.

Gleevec, see Imatinib
Idarubicin

Type: Anthracycline antitumor antibiotic.
Method of action: Intercalates between DNA base pairs and inhibits topoisomerase II, analog of daunorubicin but is more fat soluble and has increased cellular uptake.
Half-life: 14 to 35 hours (per os [PO]), 12 to 27 hours (intravenous [IV]).
Excretion: Hepatic.
Indications: Acute myeloid leukemia (AML).
Side effects: Nausea, vomiting, cardiac arrhythmias, mucositis.

Ifosfamide

Type: Synthetic nitrogen mustard alkylating agent.
Method of action: Synthetic analog of cyclophosphamide. Cross-links DNA strands and inhibits DNA and protein synthesis.
Half-life: 7 to 15 hours depending on dose.
Metabolized: Liver.
Excretion: Urine.
Indications: Testicular, breast, lung, cervical, ovarian cancers, soft-tissue sarcoma, osteosarcoma, lymphoma.
Side effects: Hemorrhagic cystitis, encephalopathy, peripheral neuropathy, renal tubular acidosis.

Imatinib (Gleevec)

Type: Monoclonal antibody to human EGFR.
Method of action: Inhibits production of Tyrosine kinase, which is a signaling molecule within the cell.
Half-life: 40 hours.
Metabolized: Liver.
Excretion: Feces.
Indications: Philadelphia chromosome-positive chronic myelogenous leukemia, gastrointestinal stromal tumor (GIST).
Side effects: Nausea, diarrhea, headaches, leg cramps, fluid retention, rash, pancytopenia with possible neutropenic infection.

Interleukin-2 (IL-2)

Type: Inflammatory cytokine, a signaling molecule to the white blood cells.

Method of action: directly effects T cell activity promoting differentiation into regulatory, effector, and memory T cells having a key role in cell-mediated immunity.

Half-life: Short.

Excretion: Urine.

Indications: Renal cell carcinoma, melanoma.

Side effects: Nausea, vomiting, flulike symptoms, rash, hypotension, diarrhea, pruritus.

• Serious: Capillary leak syndrome, cardiac toxicity, seizures, hypersensitivity.

Ipilimumab (Yervoy)

Type: Targeted T cell antibody.

Method of action: Inhibition of cytotoxic T-lymphocyte antigen 4 (CTLA-4) reducing T-regulatory cell function increasing T cell responsiveness,

Half-life: 15.4 days.

Excretion: Urine.

Indications: Metastatic malignant melanoma.

Side effects: Dermatitis, fatigue, diarrhea, pruritus, rash.

• Severe: Immune-mediated reactions including hepatitis, dermatitis, toxic epidermal necrolysis, enterocolitis, neuropathy, endocrinopathy, encephalitis.

Irinotecan

Type: Topoisomerase I inhibitor that prevents DNA from unwinding for replication.

Method of action: Carboxylesterase converts to SN-38 that has a 1,000-fold increase in chemotherapeutic effect.

Half-life: 6 to 12 hours.

Metabolized: Liver.

Excretion: Urine.

Indications: Colon cancer in FOLFIRI (5-FU, leucovorin, irinotecan).

Side effects: Diarrhea, immunosuppression, neutropenia.

Leucovorin (Folinic Acid)

Type: Thymidylate synthase inhibitor.
Method of action: Enhances effect of 5-FU.
Half-life: 6.2 hours.
Metabolized: Liver.
Excretion: Urine.
Indications: Adjunct to 5-FU for treatment of colon cancer in FOLFIRI or FOLFOX regimens.
Side effects: Enterocolitis, dehydration, diarrhea.

Methotrexate

Type: Antimetabolite and antifolate.
Method of action: Inhibits reduction of folic acid by dihydrofolate reductase.
Half-life: Dose dependent; low: 3 to 10 hours; high: 8 to 15 hours.
Metabolized: Liver.
Excretion: Urine.
Indications: Breast, head and neck, lung, bladder cancers, leukemia, lymphoma, osteosarcoma.
Side effects: Hepatotoxicity, gastric ulcers, neutropenia, pneumonitis, pulmonary fibrosis, renal failure. Neurologic damage and memory loss since it crosses blood–brain barrier.

Mitomycin C

Type: Antineoplastic antibiotic isolated from *Streptomyces* bacteria.
Method of action: Creates oxygen radicals, alkylates DNA, and forms DNA cross-linking that prevents replication; preferential for hypoxic cells.
Half-life: 48 minutes.
Metabolized: Liver.
Excretion: Urine.
Indications: Gastric and pancreatic adenocarcinoma.
Side effects: Pancytopenia, stomatitis, fatigue. Rare: pneumonitis, pulmonary fibrosis, hemolytic–uremic syndrome.

Mitoxantrone

Type: Anthracenedione antineoplastic.
Method of action: Topoisomerase II inhibitor.
Half-life: 75 hours.
Metabolized: Liver.
Excretion: Urine.
Indications: Metastatic breast cancer, prostate cancer (with prednisone), AML, NHL.
Side effects: Nausea, vomiting, alopecia, cardiotoxicity especially irreversible cardiomyopathy, immunosuppression.

Navelbine, see Vinorelbine

Nexavar, see Sorafenib

Octreotide (Sandostatin)

Type: Mimics naturally occurring somatostatin.
Method of action: Inhibits growth hormone, glucagon, insulin.
Half-life: 1.7 to 1.9 hours.
Metabolized: Liver.
Excretion: Urine.
Indications: Neuroendocrine tumors especially carcinoids and VIPomas (vasoactive intestinal peptide) causing diarrhea, flushing, hypertension.
Side effects: Headache, hypothyroidism, cardiac toxicity, gastrointestinal cramping, diarrhea/constipation, nausea, vomiting, hypoglycemia.

Ondansetron (Zofran)

Type: Antiemetic.
Method of action: Selective 5-HT3 receptor blocker in both periphery and central nervous system.
Half-life: 2 to 7 hours.
Metabolized: Liver.
Excretion: Primarily urine.
Indications: Chemotherapy-induced vomiting, prophylaxis.
Side effects: Headache, fatigue, drowsiness.

Oxaliplatin/Cisplatin/Carboplatin

Type: Platinum-based antineoplastic agents.
Method of action: Interstrand and intrastrand cross-linking of DNA leading to inability to replicate.
Half-life: 10 to 25 minutes.
Metabolized: Liver.
Excretion: Urine.
Indications: Colon cancer (as part of FOLFOX regimen with 5-FU and leucovorin), ovarian, lung, head and neck cancers.
Side effects: Peripheral neuropathy, nephrotoxicity (less so with oxaliplatin and carboplatin), fatigue, ototoxicity (hearing loss), myelosuppression (especially with carboplatin).

Paclitaxel (Taxol, Abraxane)

Type: Taxane.
Method of action: Prevents depolymerization of cellular microtubules resulting in DNA, RNA, and protein inhibition.
Half-life: 27 hours.
Metabolized: Liver.
Excretion: Fecal.
Indications: Ovarian, pancreatic, breast, non–small cell lung cancers, Kaposi's sarcoma.
Side effects: Neutropenia, alopecia, anemia, myalgia, diarrhea, leukopenia, nausea/vomiting, infection, peripheral neuropathy, mucositis, renal damage, hypotension.

Panitumumab (Vectibix)

Type: Monoclonal antibody to human EGFR.
Method of action: Binds to EGFR.
Half-life: 7.5 days.
Excretion: Systemic.
Indications: KRAS wild-type colorectal carcinoma.
Side effects: Dermatologic reaction, erythema, acneiform dermatitis, pruritus, hypomagnesemia, fatigue, abdominal pain, nausea, diarrhea/constipation, vomiting.

Pembrolizumab (Keytruda)

Type: Monoclonal antibody to PD-1 receptor.

Method of action: Binds to the PD-1 receptor and blocks its interaction with PD-L1 and PD-L2, releasing PD-1 pathway-mediated inhibition of the immune response.

Half-life: 22 days.

Excretion: Systemic.

Indications: Tumors positive for PDL-1 and not mutated EGFR or ALK genes. Usually used in melanoma, non-small cell lung cancer, head and neck squamous cell carcinoma, classical Hodgkin's lymphoma, advanced urothelial cancer, solid tumors with microsatellite instability–high (MSI-H) or a mismatch repair deficient (dMMR).

Side effects: Fatigue, pruritis, diarrhea, decreased appetite, rash, fever, cough, dyspnea, musculoskeletal pain, constipation, nausea.

Regorafenib (Stivarga)

Type: Small molecule tyrosine kinase inhibitor.Method of action: Binds to multiple tyrosine kinase receptors, antiangiogenic effect due to binding with VEGF.

Half-life: 20 to 30 hours.

Metabolized: Liver.

Excretion: Feces.

Indications: Metastatic colorectal carcinoma, advanced gastrointestinal stromal tumors.

Side effects:

- Common: Fatigue, hand–foot syndrome, diarrhea, mucositis, weight loss, infection, hypertension.
- Rare: Severe and fatal liver toxicity with bleeding, blistering of skin, myocardial infarctions, bowel perforations, severe hypertension.

Rituximab (Rituxan)

Type: Monoclonal antibody against protein CD20 found primarily on the surface of immune B cells.

Method of action: Binds with CD20 that may play a role in calcium channel regulation through the cell wall.

Half-life: 30 to 400 hours depending on dose.

Metabolized: Uncertain but potentially through reticuloendothelial cells.

Indications: Lymphomas, leukemias having predominant B cell component.

Side effects: Hypersensitivity, cardiac arrest, cytokine release syndrome, tumor lysis syndrome, pulmonary toxicity, bowel obstruction/perforation.

Sandostatin, see Octreotide
Sorafenib (Nexavar)

Type: Small molecule tyrosine kinase inhibitor.
Method of action: Binds to multiple tyrosine kinase receptors including vascular endothelial growth factor receptors (VEGFR), platelet-derived growth factor receptors (PDGFR), Raf family kinases.
Half-life: 25 to 48 hours.
Metabolized: Liver.
Excretion: Feces.
Indications: Advanced renal cell carcinoma, hepatocellular carcinoma, thyroid cancer.
Side effects:
- Very common (>10%): Hypophosphatemia, hemorrhage, rash, alopecia, diarrhea, hand–foot syndrome, hypertension, pruritus, erythema, nausea/vomiting.
- Common (1–10%): Pancytopenia, anemia, hypocalcemia, hypokalemia, depression, myocardial ischemia/infarction, congestive heart failure, renal failure.
- Rare (<1%): Hypothyroidism/hyperthyroidism, hyponatremia, dehydration, reversible posterior leukoencephalopathy, pancreatitis, gastritis, bowel perforation, anaphylaxis, angioedema, hepatitis, Stevens–Johnson syndrome, toxic epidermal necrolysis, nephrotic syndrome, rhabdomyolysis.

Stivarga, see Regorafenib
Sunitinib (Sutent)

Type: Small molecule tyrosine kinase inhibitor.
Method of action: Binds to multiple tyrosine kinase receptors including PDGFR and VEGFR, inhibits CD117 via c-kit receptor, which drives growth of gastrointestinal stromal tumor (GIST).
Half-life: 7.5 days.
Excretion: Systemic.
Indications: Renal cell carcinoma, GIST), pancreatic neuroendocrine tumors (PNET).
Side effects: Hand–foot syndrome, dermatologic toxicity, stomatitis.

Tarceva, see Erlotinib
Taxol, see Paclitaxel
Taxotere, see Docetaxel
Topotecan

Type: Topoisomerase inhibitor.
Method of action: Binds to topoisomerase I to produce double-strand breaks in DNA.
Half-life: 2 to 3 hours (IV), 3 to 6 hours (PO).
Metabolized: Liver.
Excretion: Urine, feces.
Indications: Small cell lung cancer, ovarian cancer, cervical cancer.
Side effects: Pancytopenia, nausea/vomiting, alopecia, sepsis, diarrhea, fatigue, fever, myalgia, dyspnea, rash, headache.

Vincristine

Type: Vinca alkaloid.
Method of action: Acts in M and S phases to inhibit microtubule formation inhibiting DNA and RNA synthesis.
Half-life: 10 to 155 hours.
Metabolized: Liver.
Excretion: Feces, urine.
Indications: Acute leukemia, Hodgkin's disease, NHL, Rhabdomyosarcoma, Wilms' tumor, Neuroblastoma, uveal melanoma.
Side effects: Alopecia, peripheral neuropathy, paresthesia, nephropathy, hypertension/hypotension, nausea/vomiting, myelosuppression.

Vectibix, see Panitumumab
Vinorelbine (Navelbine)

Type: Semisynthetic vinca alkaloid.
Method of action: Interferes with tubulin during mitosis.
Half-life: 28 to 44 hours.
Metabolized: Liver.
Excretion: Feces.
Indications: Non–small cell lung cancer, breast cancer, rhabdomyosarcoma.
Side effects: Peripheral neuropathy, anemia, diarrhea, nausea, asthenia, hyponatremia.

VP-16, see Etoposide
Xeloda, see Capecitabine
Yervoy, see Ipilimumab
Common Combinations of Chemotherapeutic Agents

FOLFOX: 5-FU, leucovorin, oxaliplatin for colorectal cancer.
FOLFIRI: 5-FU, leucovorin, Irinotecan for colorectal cancer.
FOLFIRINOX/FOLFOXIRI: 5-FU, leucovorin, irinotecan, oxaliplatin for advanced pancreatic cancer.
Gem/Abraxane: Gemcitabine, paclitaxel for advanced pancreatic cancer, better tolerated than FOLFIRINOX but slightly less effective.
MVAC: Methotrexate, vincristine, Adriamycin, Cytoxan for urothelial tumors.

6 Colorectal Cancer

Douglas M. Coldwell

Epidemiology

- Ten percent of new cancers in the United States and 10% of cancer mortality.
- Lifetime risk in the United States is 6%.
- Fewer than 5% inherited.
- Most sporadic and incidence dramatically increases with age.
- Occur in benign polyps that show overgrowth by epithelium and abnormal differentiation.
- Pedunculated polyps larger than 1 cm have 15% risk of progressing to cancer.
- Removal of these polyps is recommended.[1]
- Dietary factors:
  - Increased incidence with high caloric diet, red meat consumption, high saturated fats, alcohol and cigarette use, sedentary lifestyle, obesity, diabetes.
  - Decreased incidence of colon cancer with high fiber diet, antioxidant vitamins, fresh fruit and vegetable consumption, nonsteroidal anti-inflammatory use, coffee, high calcium and magnesium.[2,3]

Genetics of Colorectal Cancer

All colon cancers begin with adenomatous precursors that, when subjected to genetic mutations, progress to malignancy. Genetic mutations that activate the *WNT* signaling pathway necessary for initiation of chromosomal instability and *KRAS* (V-Ki-ras2 Kirsten rat sarcoma viral oncogene homolog) mutation with the loss of *p53* and other tumor suppressors.

About 20% of these cancers have microsatellite instability (MSI) due to defective deoxyribonucleic acid (DNA) mismatch repair gene, which is associated with *CpG* island methylation or a result of familial predisposition. Mutations occur in *KRAS*, BRAF oncogenes, *p53* tumor suppressor gene, or microsatellite containing genes that are sensitive to defective DNA mismatch repair. *BRAF* mutation is present in 10 to 20% of colorectal cancer (CRC) linked to microsatellite instability (MSI) with poorer prognosis.[4-6]

Colorectal Cancer Tumor Syndromes

- Familial adenomatous polyposis (FAP): Multiple adenomas throughout gastrointestinal (GI) tract, multiple CRC, hypertrophy of retinal epithelium.
- Gardner's syndrome: Same as FAP with desmoid tumors and mandibular osteomas.
- Turcot's syndrome: Polyposis and CRC with brain tumors, especially medulloblastoma and glioblastoma.[7]
- Hereditary nonpolyposis colorectal cancer (HNPCC or Lynch's syndrome): 70% lifetime risk of CRC with mild polyposis and presents at a younger age (<50 years old), high risk of endometrial cancer, mild risk of other GYN (gynecologic) tumors, hepatobiliary tumors, and brain tumors.[8-10]
- Peutz–Jeghers syndrome: Hamartomatous polyps throughout GI tract, mucocutaneous pigmentation, increased risk of cancer by at least ninefold.
- Cowden's disease: Multiple hamartomas in GI tract, soft tissues, thyroid, brain with increased risk of breast, uterus, thyroid, and GI cancer.[11]

Screening

Average-Risk Patient

Fecal occult blood test yearly.
Sigmoidoscopy every 5 years.
Colonoscopy every 10 years.
    There is some controversy over colonoscopy versus computed tomography (CT) colonography, but Food and Drug Administration (FDA) panel has recommended that they are equivalent for polyps 8 mm and larger with colonoscopy following immediately after CT colonography if suspicious polyps identified. Consider performing both CT and colonoscopy on the same day with the same preparation; however, this requires extensive collaboration and cooperation with the endoscopy service.

High-Risk Patient

Familial history of CRC or hereditary syndrome.
For FAP, start screening colonoscopy at age 10 years and repeat every 1 to 3 years.

For HNPCC, start screening at age 20 to 15 years.

For inflammatory bowel disease or history of polyps, screening is done every 3 to 8 years beginning from when the disease was first diagnosed.[12–14]

Staging[15]

Tumor, Node, Metastasis Staging Used

Tumor Stage

Tis = In situ adenocarcinoma confined to the glandular basement membrane or lamina propria.

T1 = Invade into but not through the submucosa.

T2 = Invade into but not through the muscularis propria.

T3 = Invade through the muscularis propria into the subserosa.

T4a = Perforate into visceral peritoneum.

T4b = Invade adjacent organs or structures.

Nodal Stage

N0 = All nodes examined are negative.

N1a = Tumor metastases in one regional lymph node (LN).

N1b = Tumor found in two or three regional LN.

N1c = Tumor found in fat around but not in lymph nodes.

N2a = Tumor in four to six regional LN.

N2b = Tumor in more than seven LN.

Metastasis Stage

M0 = No evidence of distant metastases.

M1a = Tumor in one set of distant LN or one organ.

M1b = Tumor in more than one set or distant LN or organ or peritoneum.

Residual Tumor after Resection

R0 = Histologically negative surgical margins and all LN negative.

R1 = Microscopic disease present at surgical margin.

R2 = Grossly positive margins.

Stages Due to TNM Classification

Stage 0 = Tis, N0, M0.
Stage I = T1, N0, M0 or T2, N0, M0.
Stage IIA = T3, N0, M0.
Stage IIB = T4a, N0, M0.
Stage IIC = T4b, N0, M0.
Stage IIIA = T1/T2, N1/N2a, M0.
Stage IIIB = T3/T4a, N1, M0 or T2/T3, N2a, M0 or T1/T2, N2b, M0.
Stage IIIC = T4a, N2a, M0 or T3/T4a, N2b, M0 or T4b, N1/N2, M0.
Stage IVA = T any, N any, M1a.
Stage IVB = T any, N any, M1b.

Prognosis

Stages 0, I = Tumor is completely resected and diagnosis of CRC made at pathological examination = greater than 95% 5-year survival without chemotherapy or radiation.[16]

Stages II, III = Current adjuvant chemotherapy of FOLFOX (fluorouracil/leucovorin plus oxaliplatin) = 5-year disease-free survival (DFS) of 73 to 85%, which is a statistically significant improvement over 5FULV2 (fluorouracil/leucovorin) of 67 to 68%.[17]

Stage IV = Chemotherapy using FOLFIRI (fluorouracil/leucovorin plus irinotecan) or FOLFOX = objective response rate of 55%, time to progression (TTP) = 8.4 months, overall survival (OS) from date of start of therapy = 20 to 22 months, 2-year survival of 41 to 45%. These data represent the use of chemotherapy alone without locoregional therapy.[18]

Treatment

Surgery

Complete resection of the primary is desired with R0 resection margins. Unfortunately, metastatic disease is present in 40% of patients at presentation. This is the reason that 12 to 14 LN should be sampled when surgery is performed. The presence of imaging-detected metastatic disease is usually a contraindication for surgery. However, the use of locoregional therapies, such as radioembolization, may make the tumor in the liver (the most likely site of metastases) resectable, which may be accomplished at the same time as the resection of the primary tumor. Placement of colonic stents may palliate obstructed patients until their surgery.

Chemotherapy

First-line therapy for colon cancer is now FOLFOX as adjuvant therapy after the surgical extirpation of the tumor. Since oxaliplatin causes peripheral neuropathies that may be severe, this drug may be dropped when these side effects occur. As a second-line therapy, FOLFIRI with the irinotecan supplanting the oxaliplatin is used. Other drugs may be added to FOLFOX including the following:

- Antiepidermal growth factor receptors in patients whose tumors have the wild-type KRAS gene.
- Bevacizumab, a monoclonal antibody to the vascular endothelial growth factor (VEGF) reducing the tumor vascular growth. When combined with FOLFOX, this increases progression-free survival (PFS) and OS.[19]
- Aflibercept is a molecule that traps all forms of VEGF and has a greater affinity for VEGF than do native ligands. This has resulted in an increase in PFS and OS when combined with FOLFOX.[20]
- Regorafenib, a small molecule tyrosine kinase inhibitor, is related to sorafenib. While the PFS and OS advantages were modest and the side effects of the drug were grade 3 or 4 hand–foot syndrome, hepatitis, or fatigue, its use may be considered when other forms of therapy have failed. Patients who have poor performance status, rapid progression to liver metastases, more than three liver metastases, and *KRAS* mutant have a shorter survival time.[21,22]
- When epidermal growth factor receptor (*EGFR* or *HER-1*) is activated, the production of tyrosine kinase in stimulated. Use of monoclonal antibodies such as cetuximab and panitumumab has been combined with irinotecan in previously irinotecan refractory patients who are not *KRAS* mutated, and has demonstrated an increased PFS and OS.[23,24]

Rectal Cancer

Staging

Staging criteria are the same as colon cancer (vide supra). Tumor, Node, Metastasis (TNM) classification is preferred over the older and less accurate Duke's classification. The newest change in staging rectal cancer is the recognition that both nodal status (N0 or N1) and tumor stage have independent prognostic importance.[25,26] For example, patients with

T1–2N1M0 tumors (stage III) have a better prognosis than other stage III patients, while T3N0M0 (stage II) patients have a slightly worse prognosis than the T1–2N1M0 patients.

Treatment

Stage I = Transanal resection via endoscopy for selected patients with T1 or T2 lesions whose tumor is within 8 to 10 cm of the anal verge, well or moderately well differentiated, less than 40% of the circumference of the anal wall, and have no lymphatic invasion on biopsy. It is difficult to obtain enough LN with this approach and imaging with fluorodeoxyglucose (FDG) positron emission tomography (PET) scans or magnetic resonance imaging (MRI) can be helpful. With T2 lesions, resection should be followed by adjuvant chemoradiation. Local recurrence is a problem if chemoradiation is not utilized with as many as 50% of patients' tumors recurring.[27–29]

Stages II and III = Tumors in the upper one-third of the rectum can be resected with a low anterior resection with a margin of 2 cm with a coloanal anastomosis and the patient will retain anal sphincter function. Rectal tumors in the mid or lower one-third are more problematic as they lie below the peritoneal reflection. However, the low anterior resection of the middle rectal tumors can be performed successfully, but it is highly dependent on the size of the tumor. Tumors in the lower one-third (within 6 cm of the anal verge) have traditionally been treated with an abdominal peritoneal resection where the entire rectum and anus are removed and a permanent end colostomy created. While surgery has been the primary treatment for these lesions, preoperative (neoadjuvant) chemoradiation in T3 and T4 lesions when sphincter preservation is used and in stage II/III with nodal metastases have been shown to result in less morbidity than when postoperative radiation is utilized.[30]

Stage IV = When the rectal tumor is large and has invaded the surrounding organs, the surgical approach is usually a total pelvic exenteration. While this aggressive procedure essentially removes all organs involved from the pelvis, the local recurrence rate still is approximately 33%. When an R0 resection is performed, the 5-year OS is approximately 50% when performed initially, but when recurrent disease is present it drops to 19%.[31] Careful patient selection for this extensive and morbid procedure is essential. Clinicopathologic and imaging findings can be of great assistance in predicting an R0 resection.[32]

Recurrence of Rectal Cancer

Recurrence of rectal cancer results in significant morbidity with tenesmus, intractable pain, bowel obstruction, and fistulae.

Role of Locoregional Therapy

In management of the primary tumor, external beam chemoradiation has been shown to be effective in treatment of both the primary and the nodal metastases. IR (interventional radiology) has little to no role in the initial treatment, but the recurrences may be amenable to radiofrequency ablation. If the patient presents with intractable pelvic pain, a hypogastric nerve block/ablation may assist in the management. Additionally, the use of low-dose (30 mg/m^2) cisplatinol given in the internal iliac arteries bilaterally may result in a decrease in pain. This result is not due to the response of the tumor to the chemotherapy, but the neurotoxicity of the chemotherapy.

References

1. Jemal A, Siegel R, Xu J, Ward E. Cancer statistics, 2010. CA Cancer J Clin 2010;60(5):277–300

2. Burkitt DP. Epidemiology of cancer of the colon and rectum. 1971. Dis Colon Rectum 1993;36(11):1071–1082

3. Liao X, Lochhead P, Nishihara R, et al. Aspirin use, tumor PIK3CA mutation, and colorectal-cancer survival. N Engl J Med 2012;367(17):1596–1606

4. Spring KJ, Zhao ZZ, Karamatic R, et al. High prevalence of sessile serrated adenomas with BRAF mutations: a prospective study of patients undergoing colonoscopy. Gastroenterology 2006;131(5):1400–1407

5. Toyota M, Ahuja N, Ohe-Toyota M, Herman JG, Baylin SB, Issa JP. CpG island methylator phenotype in colorectal cancer. Proc Natl Acad Sci U S A 1999;96(15):8681–8686

6. Cancer Genome Atlas Network. Comprehensive molecular characterization of human colon and rectal cancer. Nature 2012;487(7407):330–337

7. Hadjihannas MV, Brückner M, Jerchow B, Birchmeier W, Dietmaier W, Behrens J. Aberrant Wnt/beta-catenin signaling can induce chromosomal instability in colon cancer. Proc Natl Acad Sci U S A 2006;103(28):10747–10752

8. Vasen HF, Boland CR. Progress in genetic testing, classification, and identification of Lynch syndrome. JAMA 2005;293(16):2028–2030

9. Liu T, Yan H, Kuismanen S, et al. The role of hPMS1 and hPMS2 in predisposing to colorectal cancer. Cancer Res 2001;61(21):7798–7802

10. Ligtenberg MJ, Kuiper RP, Chan TL, et al. Heritable somatic methylation and inactivation of MSH2 in families with Lynch syndrome due to deletion of the 3′ exons of TACSTD1. Nat Genet 2009;41(1):112–117

11. Sweet K, Willis J, Zhou XP, et al. Molecular classification of patients with unexplained hamartomatous and hyperplastic polyposis. JAMA 2005;294(19):2465–2473

12. Sweet A, Lee D, Gairy K, Phiri D, Reason T, Lock K. The impact of CT colonography for colorectal cancer screening on the UK NHS: costs, healthcare resources and health outcomes. Appl Health Econ Health Policy 2011;9(1):51–64

13. Boone D, Halligan S, Taylor SA. Evidence review and status update on computed tomography colonography. Curr Gastroenterol Rep 2011;13(5):486–494

14. Levin B, Lieberman DA, McFarland B, et al; American Cancer Society Colorectal Cancer Advisory Group; US Multi-Society Task Force; American College of Radiology Colon Cancer Committee. Screening and surveillance for the early detection of colorectal cancer and adenomatous polyps, 2008: a joint guideline from the American Cancer Society, the US Multi-Society Task Force on Colorectal Cancer, and the American College of Radiology. Gastroenterology 2008;134(5):1570–1595

15. Edge SB, Byrd DR, Compton CC, et al. eds. AJCC Cancer Staging Manual. 7th ed. Berlin: Springer; 2010

16. Nivatvongs S. Surgical management of early colorectal cancer. World J Surg 2000;24(9):1052–1055

17. André T, Boni C, Navarro M, et al. Improved overall survival with oxaliplatin, fluorouracil, and leucovorin as adjuvant treatment in stage II or III colon cancer in the MOSAIC trial. J Clin Oncol 2009;27(19):3109–3116

18. Goldberg RM, Sargent DJ, Morton RF, et al. A randomized controlled trial of fluorouracil plus leucovorin, irinotecan, and oxaliplatin combinations in patients with previously untreated metastatic colorectal cancer. J Clin Oncol 2004;22(1):23–30

19. Saltz LB, Clarke S, Díaz-Rubio E, et al. Bevacizumab in combination with oxaliplatin-based chemotherapy as first-line therapy in metastatic colorectal cancer: a randomized phase III study. J Clin Oncol 2008;26(12):2013–2019

20. Van Cutsem E, Tabernero J, Lakomy R, et al. Addition of aflibercept to fluorouracil, leucovorin, and irinotecan improves survival in a phase III randomized trial in patients with metastatic colorectal cancer previously treated with an oxaliplatin-based regimen. J Clin Oncol 2012;30(28):3499–3506

21. Grothey A, Van Cutsem E, Sobrero A, et al; CORRECT Study Group. Regorafenib monotherapy for previously treated metastatic colorectal cancer (CORRECT): an international, multicentre, randomised, placebo-controlled, phase 3 trial. Lancet 2013;381(9863):303–312

22. Adenis A, de la Fouchardiere C, Paule B, et al. Survival, safety, and prognostic factors for outcome with Regorafenib in patients with metastatic colorectal cancer refractory to standard therapies: results from a multicenter study (REBACCA) nested within a compassionate use program. BMC Cancer 2016;16:412

23. Van Cutsem E, Köhne CH, Láng I, et al. Cetuximab plus irinotecan, fluorouracil, and leucovorin as first-line treatment for metastatic colorectal cancer: updated analysis of overall survival according to tumor KRAS and BRAF mutation status. J Clin Oncol 2011;29(15):2011–2019

24. Yamaguchi T, Iwasa S, Nagashima K, et al. Comparison of panitumumab plus irinotecan and cetuximab plus irinotecan for KRAS wild-type metastatic colorectal cancer. Anticancer Res 2016;36(7):3531–3536

25. Gunderson LL, Sargent DJ, Tepper JE, et al. Impact of T and N substage on survival and disease relapse in adjuvant rectal cancer: a pooled analysis. Int J Radiat Oncol Biol Phys 2002;54(2):386–396

26. Greene FL, Stewart AK, Norton HJ. New tumor-node-metastasis staging strategy for node-positive (stage III) rectal cancer: an analysis. J Clin Oncol 2004;22(10):1778–1784

27. Saraste D, Gunnarsson U, Janson M. Predicting lymph node metastases in early rectal cancer. Eur J Cancer 2013;49(5):1104–1108

28. Wu ZY, Zhao G, Chen Z, et al. Oncological outcomes of transanal local excision for high risk T(1) rectal cancers. World J Gastrointest Oncol 2012;4(4):84–88

29. Greenberg JA, Shibata D, Herndon JE II, Steele GD Jr, Mayer R, Bleday R. Local excision of distal rectal cancer: an update of cancer and leukemia group B 8984. Dis Colon Rectum 2008;51(8):1185–1191, discussion 1191–1194

30. Fitzgerald TL, Brinkley J, Zervos EE. Pushing the envelope beyond a centimeter in rectal cancer: oncologic implications of close, but negative margins. J Am Coll Surg 2011;213(5):589–595

31. Mohan HM, Evans MD, Larkin JO, Beynon J, Winter DC. Multivisceral resection in colorectal cancer: a systematic review. Ann Surg Oncol 2013;20(9):2929–2936

32. Chew MH, Brown WE, Masya L, Harrison JD, Myers E, Solomon MJ. Clinical, MRI, and PET-CT criteria used by surgeons to determine suitability for pelvic exenteration surgery for recurrent rectal cancers: a Delphi study. Dis Colon Rectum 2013;56(6):717–725

7 Cancer of the Pancreas

Douglas M. Coldwell

Epidemiology

- It is the 12th most prevalent cancer in the United States, and the 4th most frequent cause of cancer-related death.
- Survival rates have not significantly changed in the past 40 years.
- Patients with metastatic disease have a 5-year survival of 2%.
- Median age of onset is 71 years; 74% diagnosed between 55 and 84 years.
- Incidence in the United States is 12/100,000 with a lifetime risk of 1.5%.
- Higher incidence in smokers, exposure to chlorinated hydrocarbons, dry cleaning, and metal work, especially production of aluminum.[1,2]

Genetics

About 10% have a family history. Patients with three or more first-degree relatives having pancreatic cancer have a lifetime risk of 40%.

The *KRAS* gene is mutated in 90% of pancreatic adenocarcinomas. This gene mediates signals from growth factor receptors and the mutation overexpresses the output of the gene, increasing the growth factor signals converting it from a protooncogene to an oncogene. This occurs early in tumorigenesis. The tumor-suppressor and genome maintenance genes mutate in mid to late tumorigenesis. The *CDKN2A/p16* is mutated in over 90%, while the *TP53* and *SMAD4* genes are mutated in 75 and 55%, respectively. The latter two mutations occur in the late stages of tumor formation.[3,4]

Pathology

Pancreatic ductal adenocarcinoma demonstrates an almost universal perineural invasion, greater than most other common adenocarcinomas. Few are diagnosed early in tumorigenesis; most are diagnosed after they are beyond cure. On microscopy, a desmoplastic reaction is seen within the tumor mass, which will act to isolate the tumor cells from the chemotherapeutic agents.[5–7]

Diagnosis

Symptoms include jaundice, weight loss, abdominal pain, nausea, acholic stools, and tea-colored urine. New-onset diabetes mellitus occurs in approximately 10% of patients.[5]

Staging[8]

Tis = Carcinoma in situ.
T1 = 2 cm or less and confined to the pancreas.
T2 = Greater than 2 cm and confined to the pancreas.
T3 = Extends beyond the pancreas.
T4 = Invades visceral arteries and veins.
N0 = No regional lymph node (LN) involvement.
N1 = Regional LN metastases.
M0 = No distant metastases.
M1 = Distant metastases.
Stage 0 = Tis N0 M0.
Stage IA = T1 N0 M0 with survival (all patients) of 10 months;
    24 months with resection.
Stage IB = T2 N0 M0 with survival (all patients) of 9.1 months;
    20.6 months with resection.
Stage IIA = T3 N0 M0 with survival (all patients) of 8.1 months;
    15.4 months with resection.
Stage IIB = T1/2/3 N1 M0 with survival (all patients) of 9.7 months;
    12.7 months with resection.
Stage III = T4 N0/1 M0 with survival (all patients) of 7.7 months;
    10.6 months with resection.
Stage IV = any T any N M1 with survival (all patients) of 2.5 months;
    4.5 months with resection.

Treatment

Surgery

An R0 resection (resectable tumor) is likely if there is no abutment to either the superior mesenteric artery (SMA) or celiac axis (CA) or hepatic artery (HA) but may be abutted to the superior mesenteric vein–portal vein (SMV–PV) confluence without distortion. An R1 resection (borderline resectable) is likely if there is abutment to either the SMA or CA or there is SMV or PV distortion due to the tumor or a segment of SMV is occluded with patent vein on either side. An R2 resection (locally advanced) is likely if the tumor encases the SMA, CA, or HA, or occludes the SMV or PV without reconstruction options.[9-11]

Resection is attempted if the patient is medically fit, if there is no evidence of metastases, and if the patient is thought to have resectable disease. The surgery for right-sided lesions (those involving the head, neck, or uncinate process) is a pancreaticoduodenectomy (Whipple procedure). Those lesions on the left (tail of pancreas) are resected with a distal pancreatectomy.

Unresectable disease is due to invasion of the SMA or vein, the CA, or the SMV–PV confluence. Borderline resectable lesions are those that abut the vessels above but do not involve more than 180-degree circumference and there are potential reconstruction options available.

Chemotherapy

Adjuvant therapy is recommended using FOLFIRI (5-FU, leucovorin, irinotecan), FOLFIRINOX (5-FU, leucovorin, irinotecan, oxaliplatin for advanced pancreatic cancer) or gemcitabine monotherapies, 5-FU, or capecitabine or chemoradiation using these agents. Additional survival of 3 months is predicted from patients receiving 6 months of these therapies.

Recurrence of tumor usually occurs in the retroperitoneum, liver, peritoneum, and lung. Most patients recur at both the site of resection and distantly.

Stage III: Locally advanced disease treatment, which is unresectable.

Usually chemoradiation especially using stereotactic body radiation to limit the side effects of the treatment. Chemotherapeutic options are FOLFIRI, gemcitabine, 5-FU, or capecitabine.

Stage IV: Distant metastases.

Chemotherapy with radiation to the primary site is given as palliation. Chemotherapy can be gemcitabine ($400–500$ mg/m^2 weekly), capecitabine ($800–825$ mg/m^2 twice per day on day of radiation), or continuous infusion of 5-FU via a pump at 25 mg/m^2/d or 300 mg/m^2 on day of radiation.

Locoregional Therapy

Treatment of metastases via embolotherapy or ablation can palliate abdominal symptoms and improve quality of life, but survival is predicated on the response of the primary tumor. Due to the perineural invasion mentioned above, the tumor is likely to invade the celiac or superior mesenteric plexus, causing intractable severe pain. This pain can be treated by ablating these neural plexuses.

Treatment of the primary tumor in the operating room with irreversible electroporation has been demonstrated to shrink borderline resectable tumors or unresectable tumors, but the complications have been primarily vascular injury to the vessels, SMA or SMV, in the treated bed with hemorrhaging, pseudoaneurysm, or thrombosis.[12]

Pancreatic Neuroendocrine Tumors

Epidemiology

Pancreatic neuroendocrine tumor is more common in men than in women; age at diagnosis is 60 years. It represents only 5% of pancreatic tumors. Pancreatic ductal adenocarcinoma is 60 times more frequent than primitive neuroectodermal tumors (PNETs).

At diagnosis, 14% were localized, 22% regional disease, and 64% distant disease.

Symptoms

Related to cells of origin and hormone producing.

Most are carcinoid and, if functional, demonstrate the carcinoid syndrome after metastatic spread to the liver.

Carcinoid syndrome = Hot flashes, episodic hypertension, explosive and dehydrating diarrhea due to production of serotonin. May result in right-heart damage and mitral valve damage.

If it originates from gastrin cells, it results in parietal cell stimulation leading to hypersecretion of gastric acid causing extensive and unremitting gastric and duodenal ulcers (Zollinger–Ellison syndrome). It usually occurs in duodenum, pancreatic head, or uncinate process.

If it originates from insulin cells, it results in difficult-to-control hypoglycemia. It may occur anywhere in the pancreas. It is the most common functional PNET (30–45%).

Vasoactive intestinal peptide (VIPoma) secreting cells cause watery diarrhea, hypokalemia, and achlorhydria (Verner–Morrison syndrome).[13]

Pathology

Immunohistochemical markers to determine degree of endocrine differentiation and to determine the degree of proliferation/aggressiveness.

General markers for NET.

Neuron-specific enolase.

Chromogranin A.

Synaptophysin.

Specific markers for hormones produced by the tumoral endocrine cell.
 Proliferation rate classification is as follows:

- Grade 1 = mitotic count (MC) of less than 2 per 10 high-power field (HPF) and K_i-67 index of less than and equal to 2%.
- Grade 2 = MC of 2 to 20 per 10 HPF and Ki-67 index 3 to 20%.
- Grade 3 = MC of greater than 20 per 10 HPF and Ki-67 index greater than 20%.

Genetics

Commonly mutated genes are the following:

- *MEN1* gene is lost when the *11q13* locus is missing. Involved in epigenetic regulation. Multiple endocrine neoplasia type 1 is diagnosed when a patient with hyperparathyroidism develops either a pituitary tumor (more common in women) or a PNET usually a gastrinoma or insulinoma (more common in men) or when the *MEN1* genetic mutation is detected.
- In MEN2a, medullary thyroid cancer, primary hyperparathyroidism, and pheochromocytoma are seen together. In MEN2b, medullary thyroid cancer is associated with pheochromocytoma, marfanoid physical features, and neurofibromatosis. These syndromes are caused by a gain of function of the RET gene that has effect on the TGF-β (transforming growth factor beta) system that affects the operation of the nervous system.
- *DAXX* or *ATRX* mutations are associated with lengthening of telomeres and are chromatin-remodeling genes.
- Mammalian target of rapamycin (mTOR) pathway regulates cellular proliferation and survival through the production of tyrosine kinase. The genes include the phosphate and tensin homolog (*PTEN*), *PIK3CA*, and *TSC2*. This gene group allows the PNETs to be treated with mTOR inhibitors.[14,15]

von Hippel–Lindau syndrome includes PNETs; retinal, cerebellar, and spinal hemangioblastomas; and multiple renal cell carcinomas. The vHL gene is associated with the regulation of angiogenesis and its mutation leads to the hypervascularity of these tumors.

Tuberous sclerosis is also associated with PNETs. Since the genes *TSC-1* and *TSC-2* are normally expressed by the neuroendocrine cells and form a complex that inhibits mTOR, hamartomas and islet cell carcinomas are the most common tumors seen.

Neurofibromatosis type 1 is an autosomal-dominant mutation, which is the loss of the gene *NF1* that is associated with cutaneous neurofibromas. *NF1* has also been shown to regulate the mTOR pathway leading to tumor formation (usually somatostatinomas) in the region of the duodenum and ampulla of Vater.

Staging

Tumor

T0 = No evidence of primary tumor in pancreas.
T1 = Tumor limited to pancreas and less than and equal to 2cm.
T2 = Tumor limited to pancreas and greater than 2 cm.
T3 = Tumor extends beyond pancreas but does not involve CA or SMV.
T4 = Involves CA or SMV (unresectable).

Lymph Nodes

N0 = No regional LN involvement.
N1 = Regional LN metastases.

Metastases

M0 = No distant metastases.
M1 = Distant metastases.

Staging

Stage 0 = Tis (tumor in situ) N0 M0.
Stage IA = T1 N0 M0.
Stage IB = T2 N0 M0.
Stage IIA = T3 N0 M0.
Stage IIB = T1/2/3 N1 M0.
Stage III = T4 N0/1 M0.
Stage IV = T1/2/3/4 N0/1 M1.

Treatment

Surgery

Resection of tumors up to stage IIA should be considered if an R0 resection may be performed. If metastatic disease is present, stage IIB or III, chemotherapy should be instituted before a resection is considered since the tumor may become smaller and recede from the vessels. The goal is to maximize local disease control and increase quality of life.[16]

Chemotherapy

In tumors with grades 1 and 2 pathology, no chemotherapy and somatostatin analogues (e.g., octreotide) are used. In tumors with grade 3 pathology, platinum-based chemotherapy is usually used and is more effective when the K_i-67 index is greater than 55%.

Everolimus may also be utilized to inhibit the mTOR pathway and be combined with somatostatin analogues.

Sunitinib is a tyrosine kinase inhibitor that acts against the vascular endothelial growth factor to decrease the angiogenesis seen in PNETs.

Cytotoxic chemotherapy is controversial, but when utilized it is usually streptozocin based or dacarbazine and temozolomide based.[17]

Locoregional therapies are used in unresectable disease.

Transarterial chemoembolization (TACE) has been the standard regimen until recently due to the hypervascularity of these tumors. Superselective embolization with either drug-eluting beads or ethiodol/lipiodol has been combined with streptozocin or Adriamycin. Use of radioembolization (RE) of 90Y beads has shown a far higher rate of response (80–98%) than TACE (33–50%) with a better quality of life. However, the bilirubin must be less than 2 mg/dL to decrease the likelihood of liver failure.

Prognosis

With localized disease that is operable, mean survival is approximately 7 years, while unresectable patients with metastatic disease had an overall survival (OS) of 2.2 years. Patients with progressive disease having everolimus or sunitinib had survivals of approximately 11 months. Locoregional therapies are noted to be palliative and, while their use in these tumors has been a mainstay of therapy, increase in OS cannot be proven even though 33% of patients respond to TACE and over 80%

respond to RE. Reports of multiple sessions of RE over several years, resulting in undetectable levels of Chromogranin A, are available, suggesting that when the disease is limited to the liver, RE is a good adjunct to systemic therapy.

References

1. Bertuccio P, La Vecchia C, Silverman DT, et al. Cigar and pipe smoking, smokeless tobacco use and pancreatic cancer: an analysis from the International Pancreatic Cancer Case-Control Consortium (PanC4). Ann Oncol 2011;22(6):1420–1426

2. Andreotti G, Silverman DT. Occupational risk factors and pancreatic cancer: a review of recent findings. Mol Carcinog 2012;51(1):98–108

3. Jones S, Zhang X, Parsons DW, et al. Core signaling pathways in human pancreatic cancers revealed by global genomic analyses. Science 2008;321(5897):1801–1806

4. Yachida S, Jones S, Bozic I, et al. Distant metastasis occurs late during the genetic evolution of pancreatic cancer. Nature 2010;467(7319):1114–1117

5. Winter JM, Cameron JL, Campbell KA, et al. 1423 pancreaticoduodenectomies for pancreatic cancer: A single-institution experience. J Gastrointest Surg 2006;10(9):1199–1210, discussion 1210–1211

6. Winter JM, Maitra A, Yeo CJ. Genetics and pathology of pancreatic cancer. HPB (Oxford) 2006;8(5):324–336

7. Neesse A, Michl P, Frese KK, et al. Stromal biology and therapy in pancreatic cancer. Gut 2011;60(6):861–868

8. Edge SE, Byrd DR. AJCC Cancer Staging Manual. 7th ed. New York, NY: Springer; 2010

9. Callery MP, Chang KJ, Fishman EK, Talamonti MS, William Traverso L, Linehan DC. Pretreatment assessment of resectable and borderline resectable pancreatic cancer: expert consensus statement. Ann Surg Oncol 2009;16(7):1727–1733

10. Evans DB, Erickson BA, Ritch P. Borderline resectable pancreatic cancer: definitions and the importance of multimodality therapy. Ann Surg Oncol 2010;17(11):2803–2805

11. Varadhachary GR, Tamm EP, Abbruzzese JL, et al. Borderline resectable pancreatic cancer: definitions, management, and role of preoperative therapy. Ann Surg Oncol 2006;13(8):1035–1046

12. Schulz G, Ou J, VanMeter T, Martin RC. Early non-tumorous CT findings after irreversible electroporation of locally advanced pancreatic cancer. Abdom Imaging 2016;41(11):2142-2149.

13. Whipple AO. The surgical therapy of hyperinsulinism. J Int Chir 1938;3:237–276

14. Jiao Y, Shi C, Edil BH, et al. DAXX/ATRX, MEN1, and mTOR pathway genes are frequently altered in pancreatic neuroendocrine tumors. Science 2011;331(6021):1199–1203

15. Falconi M, Bartsch DK, Eriksson B, et al; Barcelona Consensus Conference participants. ENETS Consensus Guidelines for the management of patients with digestive neuroendocrine neoplasms of the digestive system: well-differentiated pancreatic non-functioning tumors. Neuroendocrinology 2012;95(2):120–134

16. McKenna LR, Edil BH. Update on pancreatic neuroendocrine tumors. Gland Surg 2014;3(4):258–275

17. DeVita VT, Lawrence TS, Rosenberg SA. Cancer: Principles and practice of oncology. 10th ed. Philadelphia, PA: Wolters Kluwer; 2015

8 Carcinoid Tumor (Neuroendocrine Tumors of the Gastrointestinal Tract)

Douglas M. Coldwell

Epidemiology

- 6.2 per 100,000 and rising. Found most commonly in the seventh decade of life, in males, in Caucasians, and at an advanced stage. Midgut carcinoids are more prevalent than foregut or hindgut.
- Even when small, these tumors may cause an intense local desmoplastic response and may metastasize.
  Carcinoid tumors are the second most prevalent gastrointestinal tumor.

Pathology

Arise from the neuroendocrine cells of Kulchitsky. Grading for aggressiveness is the same as for PNETs (primitive neuroectodermal tumors). Most (75%) arise in the small bowel followed in order by rectum, lung, and bronchus.[1]

Usually, the tumor is indolent with 5-year survival in 52–77% of cases.[2]

Staging

These tumors parallel that of colon carcinoma.

Diagnosis

Elevated 24-hour urine 5-HIAA (5-Hydroxyindoleacetic acid).

Elevated serum chromogranin A.

Computed tomography or magnetic resonance imaging demonstrating a mass in the small bowel or colon, with or without liver metastases.

Somatostatin receptor-based scintigraphy (OctreoScan).

Carcinoid syndrome

It usually occurs with midgut carcinoid tumor metastases to the liver or to organs that do not supply the portal vein, for example, ovary, due to release of tumor-derived factors such as serotonin, dopamine, tachykinins, histamine, and prostaglandins.

Some of the symptoms include diarrhea, flushing, wheezing, carcinoid heart disease, episodic hypertension. Flushing is most common (94% of patients) and occurs in the upper chest, head, and neck. It may be provoked by alcohol, nuts, cheese, and stress. Diarrhea is present in 80% of cases. Heart disease involves carcinoid plaques in the tricuspid and pulmonary valves due to the serotonin released by the tumor in the liver. Valve lesions may lead to right-sided heart failure.

All patients undergoing any procedure should be blocked with octreotide (100–500 µg) intravenously 1 to 2 hours before the procedure.[3] Patients who do not respond to somatostatin may benefit from interferon α.[4]

Treatment

Surgery

Surgery for debulking if the tumor has not metastasized. Liver resection of metastatic disease can improve the 5-year survival from 36 to 61% compared with historical controls.[5–7]

Chemotherapy

Long-acting octreotide given subcutaneously inhibits tumor growth so that 50% of patients have shrinkage of liver metastases by inhibiting VEGF (vascular endothelial growth factor) and angiogenesis. Patients with a resected primary and low hepatic tumor burden appear to benefit most from octreotide therapy.

mTOR (mammalian target of rapamycin) inhibitors such as everolimus and angiogenesis inhibitors such as bevacizumab have each shown about a 30% response rate. Research into combinations of these drugs with octreotide is ongoing.[8,9]

Locoregional Therapies

Transarterial chemoembolization (TACE) and embolotherapy have been the backbone of treatment for metastatic carcinoid to the liver. Symptomatic response to therapy has been between 67 and 100% with median survival of 31 months. However, this is complicated by the postembolization syndrome and hospitalization for 2 to 4 days to manage the nausea, vomiting, pain, and liver function test (LFT) elevation. Carcinoid syndrome is palliated by TAE (transarterial embolization) or TACE with a response rate of 84% with decreasing the elevated 5-HIAA markers with excellent palliation of symptoms. Radioembolization is becoming the procedure of choice for locoregional therapy of these lesions. The response rate increases to 50 to 90% with mean survival of at least 70 months. While this intra-arterial therapy is palliative, carcinoid tumors are usually indolent in their growth and extremely hypervascular; locoregional therapy is preferred as second-line therapy after octreotide therapy since any use of angiogenesis-inhibiting drugs will make the neovascularity less of a target for this therapy.[10,11]

Isolated, countable[1-5] metastases in the liver can also be treated by ablative therapies, such as radiofrequency ablation, ethanol injection, microwave, or irreversible electroporation, and show an excellent sustained response when the tumor is less than 3 cm in diameter.

References

1. Modlin IM, Lye KD, Kidd M. A 5-decade analysis of 13,715 carcinoid tumors. Cancer 2003;97(4):934–959

2. Soga J. Early-stage carcinoids of the gastrointestinal tract: an analysis of 1914 reported cases. Cancer 2005;103(8):1587–1595

3. Kvols LK, Moertel CG, O'Connell MJ, Schutt AJ, Rubin J, Hahn RG. Treatment of the malignant carcinoid syndrome. Evaluation of a long-acting somatostatin analogue. N Engl J Med 1986;315(11):663–666

4. Tiensuu Janson EM, Ahlström H, Andersson T, Oberg KE. Octreotide and interferon alfa: a new combination for the treatment of malignant carcinoid tumours. Eur J Cancer 1992;28A(10):1647–1650

5. McEntee GP, Nagorney DM, Kvols LK, Moertel CG, Grant CS. Cytoreductive hepatic surgery for neuroendocrine tumors. Surgery 1990;108(6):1091–1096

6. Sarmiento JM, Heywood G, Rubin J, Ilstrup DM, Nagorney DM, Que FG. Surgical treatment of neuroendocrine metastases to the liver: a plea for resection to increase survival. J Am Coll Surg 2003;197(1):29–37

7. Sarmiento JM, Que FG. Hepatic surgery for metastases from neuroendocrine tumors. Surg Oncol Clin N Am 2003;12(1):231–242

8. Yao JC, Shah MH, Ito T, et al; RAD001 in Advanced Neuroendocrine Tumors, Third Trial (RADIANT-3) Study Group. Everolimus for advanced pancreatic neuroendocrine tumors. N Engl J Med 2011;364(6):514–523

9. Raymond E, Dahan L, Raoul JL, et al. Sunitinib malate for the treatment of pancreatic neuroendocrine tumors. N Engl J Med 2011;364(6):501–513

10. Gupta S, Yao JC, Ahrar K, et al. Hepatic artery embolization and chemoembolization for treatment of patients with metastatic carcinoid tumors: the M.D. Anderson experience. Cancer J 2003;9(4):261–267

11. Gupta S. Intra-arterial liver-directed therapies for neuroendocrine hepatic metastases. Semin Intervent Radiol 2013;30(1):28–38

9 Hepatocellular Carcinoma

Douglas M. Coldwell

Epidemiology

Overall, hepatocellular carcinoma (HCC) is the fifth most common cancer in the world and the second most common cause of cancer death in the world. It is the fifth most common cancer in men and seventh in women worldwide. Causes are well known with hepatitis B and hepatitis C (HCV) and ethanol abuse causing cirrhosis leading to the formation of HCC in approximately 10 years. Asian and sub-Saharan Africa rates are declining due to hepatitis immunization but U.S. rates are rapidly increasing due to immigration from high incidence areas as well as increasing drug abuse resulting in HCV infection.[1]

Pathology

Genetics

HCC is caused by alterations in 140 genes belonging to 12 signaling pathways that regulate core cellular processes. New microarray technology will be able to pinpoint more specific "druggable" mutations.[2] Not only the genetic alterations, but also the epigenetic alterations such as DNA methylation are being studied. These changes are thought to be early events in the evolution of HCC. The global hypomethylation can be categorized as to the origin of the HCC and correlate well with subsets of patients.[3,4] HCC develops on a background of chronic liver disease and more than 80% demonstrate cirrhosis. *Beta-catenins* and *TP53* are the most frequently mutated oncogene and tumor suppressor genes in HCC.[5,6] A low-grade dysplastic nodule develops in the cirrhotic liver, which then undergoes oxidative stress and transforms into a high-grade dysplastic nodule. With progressive activation of adverse signaling pathways and immune response, this high-grade nodule becomes an early HCC and begins proliferation. This is progressive loss of differentiation and activates the *Myc* gene, *Pi3K* (phosphoinositide-3 kinase) and TGF-β (transforming growth factor-β) signaling, and epithelial mesenchymal transition with metastases development.[7,8]

Staging[9]

Tumor

T1 = Solitary tumor without vascular invasion.
T2 = Solitary tumor with vascular invasion or multiple tumors less than 5cm in diameter.
T3a = Multiple tumors greater than 5cm in diameter.
T3b = Tumor involving major branch of the portal or hepatic veins.
T4 = Tumor with direct invasion of adjacent organs or perforation of visceral peritoneum.

Lymph Nodes

N0 = No regional lymph node (LN) metastasis.
N1 = Regional LN metastasis.

Metastases

M0 = No distant metastasis.
M1 = Distant metastasis.
Stage I = T1 N0 M0.
Stage II = T2 N0 M0.
Stage IIIA = T3a N0 M0.
Stage IIIB = T3b N0 M0.
Stage IIIC = T4 N0 M0.
Stage IVA = T1/2/3/4 N1 M0.
Stage IVB = any T any N M1.

Treatment

Untreated HCC has a 5-year survival of less than 10%.

Surgery

Liver resection is preferred for patients with noncirrhotic HCC or with Child–Pugh A patients. Patients with a greater degree of liver dysfunction are not candidates since they do not have enough normal hepatocytes to maintain normal function. After liver resection, the patient needs to have at least 30% of the volume of the normal liver to maintain normal function. If this fraction is borderline, the portal vein (PV) of the segments to be resected may be embolized with particles and coils to shift the flow of the PV to the anticipated remnant fraction. The PV is accessed transhepatically, then each segment is to be removed and embolized with particles and coils. This procedure will enlarge the remnant fraction by 5 to 15% and may allow the HCC to be resected.[10,11] The 5-year survival of resected HCC is between 50 and 60% with perioperative mortality around 2 to 7%.[12,13] The two prognostic factors associated with improved survival are lower T stage with smaller tumor size and an R0 resection with a 2-cm margin. The larger the HCC, the more likely it is that satellite tumors are present in the liver; a 2-cm margin is difficult to obtain and micrometastatic disease will likely be present. Without clear margins and a 2-cm tumor-free area around the tumor, the likelihood of recurrence as well as development of metastatic disease is increased.[14]

Transplant

Model for End-Stage Liver Disease

The Model for End-Stage Liver Disease (MELD) scores[15] = 3.78 × b_bilirubin (mg/dL) + 11.2 × INR + 9.57 × creatinine (mg/dL) + 6.43 × etiology (cholestatic or alcoholic, 0; otherwise, 1).
The UNOS (United Network for Organ Sharing) modification is as follow[16]:
If dialyzed twice in 7 days, creatinine = 4.0.
Any value less than 1, rounded up to 1.
MELD scores predict mortality at 3 months:

- ≥ 40 = 70%.
- 30–39 = 53%.
- 20–29 = 20%.
- 10–19 = 6%.
- ≤9 = 2%.

The scores are used as one criterion for priority on transplant list.

Milan Criteria[17]

Transplant for HCC is used if there is only one lesion less than and equal to 5cm or one to three lesions each less than and equal to 3cm.
Locoregional therapy can limit the dropout from the transplant list due to progressive disease by utilizing ethanol injection, ablative

therapies, embolotherapies to include bland, chemoembolization and radioembolization. In T1 and T2 HCC, there is a 95% tumor-free survival after transplant after 4 years.[18]

If the patient is not a transplant candidate and there are no metastases, local ablation with percutaneous ethanol injection, radiofrequency, or microwave ablation can be utilized to treat the lesions if less than 4 cm in diameter and are few in number (every interventional radiologist has their own definition of few but it is usually less than 6). For lesions less than 5cm in diameter and patients fulfilling the Milan criteria, RFA of the lesions was compared with surgical resection. The 1-, 3-, 5-year survivals for resection are 93, 73, and 64%, respectively, while for RFA, the results are 96, 71, and 68%, respectively.[19] For smaller HCCs, this study along with others suggests that similar results may be obtained from adequate ablation of these tumors rather than surgical resection.

For more advanced lesions, palliative therapy is primarily arterial embolization. Response to bland and chemoembolization is approximately the same at 50% for tumor shrinkage and stabilization, but the overall survival at 3 years is 10 to 40%. For radioembolization, the response rate is between 75 and 90% with overall survival of 2 years with a 3-year survival of 30 to 50%.[20] Embolotherapy is being utilized to address gross disease as a cytoreductive therapy and combine it with sorafenib. In patients who are stage IV, symptomatic therapy with embolization and celiac plexus ablation is combined with sorafenib with an expected survival of less than 3 months.

Chemotherapy

Until recently, there was no active chemotherapy drug available. Doxorubicin was previously used, but its response rate of 15% was not significant. In 2007, the SHARP trial demonstrated the efficacy of sorafenib in HCC with a 44% improvement in overall survival when compared with placebo and a median survival and time to progression was improved by 3 months each.[21] Other chemotherapeutic approaches that have shown to be of interest are bevacizumab alone, bevacizumab with erlotinib, and gemcitabine with oxaliplatin. All of these chemotherapeutic regimens have a response rate of approximately 20% and an overall survival of a year.[22]

Fibrolamellar Hepatocellular Cancer

This is a rare variant of HCC. It is slow growing, seen in younger patients peaking in the third decade, not usually associated with HCV or cirrhosis. A higher percentage (>15%) of patients present with LN involvement. Surgery is accepted as first-line treatment when resection is possible. If the tumor is unresectable, a liver transplant should be considered since the 1-, 3-, and 5-year survivals are 90, 75, and 38%, respectively.[23,24] Most patients present with stage IV disease with a median survival of almost 7 years.[25]

References

1. El-Serag HB. Epidemiology of viral hepatitis and hepatocellular carcinoma. Gastroenterology 2012;142(6):1264–1273.e1

2. Vogelstein B, Papadopoulos N, Velculescu VE, Zhou S, Diaz LA Jr, Kinzler KW. Cancer genome landscapes. Science 2013;339(6127):1546–1558

3. Feinberg AP, Ohlsson R, Henikoff S. The epigenetic progenitor origin of human cancer. Nat Rev Genet 2006;7(1):21–33

4. Calvisi DF, Ladu S, Gorden A, et al. Mechanistic and prognostic significance of aberrant methylation in the molecular pathogenesis of human hepatocellular carcinoma. J Clin Invest 2007;117(9):2713–2722

5. Cleary SP, Jeck WR, Zhao X, et al. Identification of driver genes in hepatocellular carcinoma by exome sequencing. Hepatology 2013;58(5):1693–1702

6. Kan Z, Zheng H, Liu X, et al. Whole-genome sequencing identifies recurrent mutations in hepatocellular carcinoma. Genome Res 2013;23(9):1422–1433

7. Karin M. Nuclear factor-kappaB in cancer development and progression. Nature 2006;441(7092):431–436

8. Luedde T, Schwabe RF. NF-κB in the liver—linking injury, fibrosis and hepatocellular carcinoma. Nat Rev Gastroenterol Hepatol 2011;8(2):108–118

9. Edge SB, Compton CC. The American Joint Committee on Cancer: the 7th edition of the AJCC cancer staging manual and the future of TNM. Ann Surg Oncol 2010;17(6):1471–1474

10. Clavien PA, Petrowsky H, DeOliveira ML, Graf R. Strategies for safer liver surgery and partial liver transplantation. N Engl J Med 2007;356(15):1545–1559

11. Capussotti L, Ferrero A, Viganò L, Polastri R, Tabone M. Liver resection for HCC with cirrhosis: surgical perspectives out of EASL/AASLD guidelines. Eur J Surg Oncol 2009;35(1):11–15

12. Yang LY, Fang F, Ou DP, Wu W, Zeng ZJ, Wu F. Solitary large hepatocellular carcinoma: a specific subtype of hepatocellular carcinoma with good outcome after hepatic resection. Ann Surg 2009;249(1):118–123

13. Wang J, Xu LB, Liu C, Pang HW, Chen YJ, Ou QJ. Prognostic factors and outcome of 438 Chinese patients with hepatocellular carcinoma underwent partial hepatectomy in a single center. World J Surg 2010;34(10):2434–2441

14. Lise M, Bacchetti S, Da Pian P, Nitti D, Pilati PL, Pigato P. Prognostic factors affecting long term outcome after liver resection for hepatocellular carcinoma: results in a series of 100 Italian patients. Cancer 1998;82(6):1028–1036

15. Kamath PS, Wiesner RH, Malinchoc M, et al. A model to predict survival in patients with end-stage liver disease. Hepatology 2001;33(2):464–470

16. UNOS. MELD/PELD calculator documentation. www.unos.org/wp-content/uploads/unos/MELD_PELD_Calculator_Documentation.pdf. Accessed August 15, 2016

17. Mazzaferro V, Regalia E, Doci R, et al. Liver transplantation for the treatment of small hepatocellular carcinomas in patients with cirrhosis. N Engl J Med 1996;334(11):693–699

18. Lubienski A. Hepatocellular carcinoma: interventional bridging to liver transplantation. Transplantation 2005;80(1, Suppl):S113–S119

19. Chen MS, Li JQ, Zheng Y, et al. A prospective randomized trial comparing percutaneous local ablative therapy and partial hepatectomy for small hepatocellular carcinoma. Ann Surg 2006;243(3):321–328

20. Llovet JM, Real MI, Montaña X, et al; Barcelona Liver Cancer Group. Arterial embolisation or chemoembolisation versus symptomatic treatment in patients with unresectable hepatocellular carcinoma: a randomised controlled trial. Lancet 2002;359(9319):1734–1739

21. Llovet JM, Ricci S, Mazzaferro V, et al; SHARP Investigators Study Group. Sorafenib in advanced hepatocellular carcinoma. N Engl J Med 2008;359(4):378–390

22. Kaseb AO, Garrett-Mayer E, Morris JS, et al. Efficacy of bevacizumab plus erlotinib for advanced hepatocellular carcinoma and predictors of outcome: final results of a phase II trial. Oncology 2012;82(2):67–74

23. Pinna AD, Iwatsuki S, Lee RG, et al. Treatment of fibrolamellar hepatoma with subtotal hepatectomy or transplantation. Hepatology 1997;26(4):877–883

24. El-Gazzaz G, Wong W, El-Hadary MK, et al. Outcome of liver resection and transplantation for fibrolamellar hepatocellular carcinoma. Transpl Int 2000;13(Suppl 1):S406–S409

25. Ang CS, Kelley RK, Choti MA, et al. Clinicopathologic characteristics and survival outcomes of patients with fibrolamellar carcinoma: data from the fibrolamellar carcinoma consortium. Gastrointest Cancer Res 2013;6(1):3–9

10 Cholangiocarcinoma

Douglas M. Coldwell

Epidemiology

Predisposing Factors

Predisposing factors of cholangiocarcinoma (CCA) include cirrhosis, Hepatitis B and C, human immunodeficiency virus (HIV), choledochal cyst, chronic calculi of the intrahepatic and extrahepatic bile ducts, primary sclerosing cholangitis, parasites (*Clonorchis sinensis* and *Opisthorchis viverrini*). All of these result in chronic inflammation of the biliary tract. Many are also implicated in the formation of hepatocellular carcinoma (HCC).

Approximately 2,500 new cases of intrahepatic CCA (iCCA) occur in the United States each year. Incidence increases with age with most patients presenting over 65 years of age. However, patients having choledochal cysts and primary sclerosing cholangitis present in their 40s. There is a slight male predominance. This tumor is most common in Hispanics and least common in African Americans.[1,2]

Pathology

iCCA occurs peripherally to the second-order bile ducts. Distal extrahepatic CCA (dCCA) arises from the common hepatic duct to the ampulla. Perihilar CCA (pCCA) arises between the second-order bile ducts and the common hepatic ducts.

Gross pathology is either mass forming, periductal infiltrating, or sclerosing, which results in a highly desmoplastic response to the tumor with extensive fibrosis containing scattered tumor cells. Most (95%) are adenocarcinomas.[3]

Differential diagnosis includes HCC and metastatic colon cancer. Immunohistochemical findings of staining positively for CA19-9 or carcinoembryonic antigen (CEA) may differentiate from HCC. Positive staining for cytokeratin 7 implicates biliary origin and cytokeratin 20 is focal and rare in iCCA while diffusely positive in colon adenocarcinomas. Serum CA19-9 levels are usually elevated.

Genetics

Since it appears that most are due to inflammation, IL-6, inducible nitric oxide synthase (*iNOS*), and cyclooxygenase 2 (*COX-2*) are involved. The genetics are less clear than many other tumors due to its rarity, and the results for iCCA, dCCA, and pCCA have been combined in most research.[4]

Diagnosis

iCCA: It may be asymptomatic but there are often complaints of RUQ (right upper quadrant) pain/mass or weight loss. Jaundice occurs late due to infiltration of the liver by tumor.

dCCA and pCCA: Painless obstructive jaundice occurs early.

The treatment and survival of CCA are due to the location in the biliary tree that the cancer originates and its stage and operability on presentation.[5]

Staging for Intrahepatic Cholangiocarcinoma[6]

Tumor

- T0 = No evidence of primary tumor.
- Tis = Tumor in situ.
- T1 = Solitary tumor without vascular invasion.
- T2a = Solitary tumor with vascular invasion.
- T2b = Multiple tumors with or without vascular invasion.
- T3 = Tumor perforating the visceral peritoneum or direct invasion into local extrahepatic structures.
- T4 = Periductal invasion.

Lymph Nodes

- N0 = No regional lymph nodes involved.
- N1 = Regional lymph nodes involved.

Metastases

- M0 = No distant metastases.
- M1 = Distant metastases present.

Staging

- Stage 0 = Tis N0 M0.
- Stage I = T1 N0 M0.
- Stage II = T2 N0 M0.
- Stage III = T3 N0 M0.
- Stage IVa = T4 N0 M0 or any T, N1 M0.
- Stage IVb = any T, any N, M1.

Treatment

Surgery

Indications for surgery are not as clear in this disease as the extent of disease is not necessarily clearly depicted by the cross-sectional imaging studies. With limited disease, an R0 resection may be obtained; however, without a complete resection, the lymph node status, positive margins, and vascular invasion are significant prognostic indicators, as are a serum CA19-9 level greater than 1,000 mg/dL and tumor size.[7,8]

Stage I: An R0 resection can usually be obtained in iCCA and with adjuvant chemotherapy, 5-year survival is approximately 60%, but an R0 resection can be obtained in only approximately 30% of patients. Liver transplantation is not an option as the survival is 29% at 5 years.[9]

Stage II: R1 or R2 resection with adjuvant chemotherapy; 5-year survival is approximately 20% since there are also nodal metastases.

Stage III:

Intrahepatic disease only: Locoregional therapy with adjuvant chemotherapy. Median survival is 20 months for transarterial chemoembolization (TACE) and 44 months for radioembolization (RE).[10]

Extrahepatic disease: Chemotherapy only. Median survival is 15 months.

Stage IV: Chemotherapy only. Median survival is 12 months.

Chemotherapy

Current standard of care is a combination of gemcitabine at 1,000 mg/m^2 with cisplatin at 25 mg/m^2 given intravenously on days 1 and 8 every 21 days for 6 months. Median survival is approximately 12 months with a progression-free survival of 8 months and a response rate of 26%.

Locoregional

The use of TACE and RE in patients with stage III disease in combination with adjuvant chemotherapy doubles their survival. However, According to The Eastern Cooperative Oncology Group (ECOG), 0–1 patients should only be treated with intra-arterial (IA) modalities, as the side effects may be of more consequence than the benefits in less healthy patients. Nevertheless, palliative locoregional therapy may address the abdominal pain and lethargy that is common in liver tumor patients. Use of ablative techniques such as radiofrequency ablation, microwave ablation, irreversible electroporation, or ethanol injection may be of assistance in controlling limited disease in the liver.

Staging for Perihilar Cholangiocarcinoma[6,11,12]

Tumor

- T0 = No evidence of primary tumor.
- Tis = Tumor in situ.
- T1 = Tumor confined to the bile duct with extension up to the muscle layer or fibrous tissue.
- T2a = Tumor invades beyond the wall of the bile duct to adjacent adipose tissue.
- T2b = Tumor invades adjacent hepatic parenchyma.
- T3 = Tumor invades unilateral branches of portal vein or hepatic artery.
- T4 = Tumor invades main portal vein, common hepatic artery, or branches of either bilaterally.

Lymph Nodes

- N0 = No regional lymph nodes involved.
- N1 = Regional lymph nodes involved.
- N2 = Metastases to nodes outside of regional, for example, periaortic, pericaval, etc.

Metastases

- M0 = No distant metastases.
- M1 = Distant metastases present.

Staging

- Stage 0 = Tis N0 M0.
- Stage I = T1 N0 M0.
- Stage II = T2a/T2b N0 M0.
- Stage IIIA = T3 N0 M0.
- Stage IIIB = T1–3 N1 M0.
- Stage IVA = T4 N0, N1 M0 or any T, N1 M0.
- Stage IVb = any T, N2, M0 or any T, any N, M1.

Treatment

Surgery

In early-stage pCCA, complete excision of the tumor may require a complete hepatectomy if the lesion is near the junction of the bile ducts. This would require liver transplantation if there was no extrahepatic disease demonstrated on magnetic resonance imaging (MRI), or endoscopy and organs were available for a suitable transplant candidate as defined by local transplant standards. In a select group of patients, this has been shown to have a 5-year survival rate of 53% and a 65% recurrence-free survival rate.[13] In other early-stage pCCA patients, resection should be performed with adjuvant chemotherapy. With an R0 resection, the 5-year survival rate is 11 to 43%, while with an R1 or R2 resection and N1 disease, the survival rate is 0%. In unresectable patients, either chemotherapy alone with gemcitabine and cisplatin as described earlier, or chemoradiation using 5-fluorouracil as a radiation sensitizer with external beam radiotherapy, the 5-year survival is less than 5% with median survival of 12 months.[12]

Chemotherapy

The gemcitabine–cisplatin regimen described earlier is again recommended for this type of CCA.

Palliation

pCCA is most likely to be unresectable and the patients face obstruction of the biliary ducts with significant loss of quality of life. Placement of covered metallic stents, either by endoscopy or by percutaneous means, should only be attempted in those patients with less than 6 months of expected survival as the stents can become narrowed or obstructed at about 6 months. Covered stents have a longer patency since the covering will resist tumor infiltration. If such a stent is used, it should extend beyond the tumor by at least 1 cm on each end. Otherwise, a patient with good performance status can be effectively palliated with either plastic stents placed by endoscopy that require regular changes with endoscopy or percutaneous stents that only require an outpatient visit to the interventional radiology department. Such internal–external stents should be flushed regularly (about once per week) with sterile saline and changed every 2 to 3 months.[14]

Staging for Distal Cholangiocarcinoma[6]

Tumor

- T0 = No evidence of primary tumor.
- Tis = Tumor in situ.
- T1 = Tumor confined to the bile duct histologically.
- T2a = Tumor invades beyond the wall of the bile duct.
- T3 = Tumor invades adjacent organs without involvement of celiac axis or superior mesenteric artery.
- T4 = Tumor invades celiac axis or superior mesenteric artery.

Lymph Nodes

- N0 = No regional lymph nodes involved.
- N1 = Regional lymph nodes involved.

Metastases

- M0 = No distant metastases.
- M1 = Distant metastases present.

Staging

- Stage 0 = Tis N0 M0.
- Stage IA = T1 N0 M0.
- Stage IB = T2 N0 M0.
- Stage IIA = T3 N0 M0.
- Stage IIB = T1–3 N1 M0.
- Stage III = T4, any N0, M0.
- Stage IV = any T, any N, M1.

Treatment

Surgery

Resection is more likely in dCCA with an improved response rate when compared with pCCA. Early-stage dCCA (stages IA–IIA) should be operated upon and an R0 resection performed. With adjuvant therapy, a 5-year survival of 27% with a mean of 25 months is expected. With an R1 or R2 resection with N1 disease (stage IIB) with adjuvant chemotherapy, the 5-year survival is still 27%. With unresectable disease or metastatic disease, either chemotherapy or chemoradiation may be utilized with expected 5-year survivals of less than 5% with a median survival of approximately 12 months.[15,16]

Locoregional Therapy

The pCCA and dCCA are amenable to palliation of their obstructive symptoms by internal–external stenting or placement of a metal stent as described earlier. Additionally, brachytherapy using iridium wires is a possibility through the drainage catheter tracts. This therapy has shown some promise in local disease mitigation.

Gallbladder Cancer

Epidemiology

The presence of chronic cholelithiasis is the single best prognostic factor in the diagnosis of gallbladder cancer (GBC). This tumor occurs most frequently in patients over 65 years who have had cholelithiasis for at least 10 years. The incidence of GBC is stabilizing or declining in those countries where the use of laparoscopic cholecystectomy has become accepted and prevalent. Other risk factors include calcification of the gallbladder wall, anomalous pancreatic biliary duct junction, choledochal cysts, environmental exposures, and *Salmonella typhi* carriers since the carriers also have a chronic inflammation of the gallbladder wall.[17–20]

Pathology

Most GBC occur in the fundus (60%), then in the body (30%) and fewest in the neck (10%) of the GB. It has a propensity to spread to adjacent organs, seed the peritoneal lining, and along needle biopsy paths. Most are adenocarcinomas and are infiltrative. Other forms of GBC are papillary, which is confined to the lumen of the GB, and nodular. Nodular GBC forms large masses and invades the adjacent liver. At autopsy, almost all patients have lymphatic spread (94%), most have hematogenous metastases (65–82%), and 60% have peritoneal carcinomatosis.[21] While gallstones are not a prerequisite for GBC, they are found in 75% of patients. Anomalous pancreatic biliary duct junctions such as a choledochal cyst are prone to GBC and other biliary tract cancers and acquire them at an earlier age. CA19-9 levels greater than 20 U/mL are diagnostic of GBC in 80%.[22]

Genetics

KRAS and *p53* mutations are frequently found. Mutant *p53* is almost universally found in invasive carcinomas and is less common the more normal the histology becomes. The malignant potential of anomalous pancreatic biliary junction has been determined to be very high and is associated with premalignant histologic changes of epithelial hyperplasia with papillary or villous appearance. Even the nonmalignant portions of the GB in patients with anomalous pancreaticobiliary junction (APBJ) associated GBCA demonstrate hyperplastic changes that are much more evident than those seen in patients without APBJ.[23]

Staging[6]

Tumor

- Tis = Found only in epithelial layer of the gallbladder, in situ.
- T1a = Tumor penetrates the lamina propria.
- T1b = Tumor penetrates the muscularis.
- T2 = Tumor penetrates into perimuscular fibrous tissue.
- T3 = Tumor grown through the serosa or has invaded adjacent liver or nearby structure.
- T4 = Tumor has invaded portal vein or hepatic vein or grown into two or more structures outside the liver.

Lymph Nodes

- N0 = Not spread to nodes.
- N1 = Tumor in adjacent nodes.
- N2 = Tumor in distant nodes, for example, along the aorta, vena cava, or celiac axis.

Metastases

- M0 = no distant metastases.
- M1 = distant metastases present.

Stages

- Stage 0 = Tis, N0, M0.
- Stage 1= T1, N0, M0.
- Stage II = T2, N0, M0.
- Stage IIIA = T3, N0, M0.
- Stage IIIB = T1–3, N1, M0.
- Stage IVA = Any T, N2, M0.
- Stage IVB = Any T, any N, M1.

Treatment

Surgery

Stages I, II, and some IIIs may be resectable, but few GBC found at presentation are resectable to R0. Thus the treatment is primarily based on chemotherapy and radiation.

Chemotherapy

The combination of gemcitabine and cisplatin is considered to be the standard of care. The treatment is similar to CCA and eventually, genetic markers will dictate the treatments utilized.

Radiation

For patients receiving 5-FU plus external beam radiation therapy to a median dose of 54 Gy as adjunct therapy, patients having gross residual tumor, the median survival was 0.6 year, with a 2-year control rate of 0%. In comparison, patients with microscopic residual tumor had median survival of 1.4 years and a 2-year control rate of 80%. Those patients having no residual tumor had a median survival of 15.1 years with a 2-year control rate of 88%.[24] Patients having greater than 54 Gy had a 100% 3-year local control rate, while those with less than 54 Gy had a 65% rate.[25]

Prognosis

Five-year survival rates with an R0 resection (negative surgical margins):

- Stage I: 90%.
- Stage II: 80%.
- Stage III: 40%.
- Stage IV: 15%.

In resectable patients with stage I or II disease, the 5-year survival varied between 15 and 90% depending on the surgery and radiotherapy received. In stages III and IV, the 1-year survival rate is less than 5%.[26,27]

Role for Interventional Radiology

Biopsy with a fine needle can be performed, but the possibility of seeding along the needle path should be considered a relative contraindication. As with most biliary tract tumors, management of biliary obstruction via internal–external stents or internal-covered stents can be utilized. Since the prognosis is so devastating, use of embolotherapy can provide symptomatic relief as well as the possibility of tumor shrinkage. The use of IA delivery of a chemotherapy agent has been utilized with some success when combined with radiation. In a report, 27 patients were treated with IA mitomycin C. The response rate of the IA patients was 48% with a median survival for responders of 34 months and for nonresponders of 8 months. The survival after IA therapy was 14 months in responders and 4 month in nonresponders.[28]

References

1. Patel T. Cholangiocarcinoma—controversies and challenges. Nat Rev Gastroenterol Hepatol 2011;8(4):189–200

2. Razumilava N, Gores GJ. Classification, diagnosis, and management of cholangiocarcinoma. Clin Gastroenterol Hepatol 2013;11(1):13–21.e1, quiz e3–e4

3. Martin RC, Klimstra DS, Schwartz L, Yilmaz A, Blumgart LH, Jarnagin W. Hepatic intraductal oncocytic papillary carcinoma. Cancer 2002;95(10):2180–2187

4. Sia D, Tovar V, Moeini A, Llovet JM. Intrahepatic cholangiocarcinoma: pathogenesis and rationale for molecular therapies. Oncogene 2013;32(41):4861–4870

5. Choi BI, Han JK, Shin YM, Baek SY, Han MC. Peripheral cholangiocarcinoma: comparison of MRI with CT. Abdom Imaging 1995;20(4):357–360

6. Edge SB, Compton CC. The American Joint Committee on Cancer: the 7th edition of the AJCC cancer staging manual and the future of TNM. Ann Surg Oncol 2010;17(6):1471–1474

7. Nakanuma Y, Sasaki M, Ishikawa A, Tsui W, Chen TC, Huang SF. Biliary papillary neoplasm of the liver. Histol Histopathol 2002;17(3):851–861

8. Poultsides GA, Zhu AX, Choti MA, Pawlik TM. Intrahepatic cholangiocarcinoma. Surg Clin North Am 2010;90(4):817–837

9. Ribero D, Pinna AD, Guglielmi A, et al; Italian Intrahepatic Cholangiocarcinoma Study Group. Surgical approach for long-term survival of patients with intrahepatic cholangiocarcinoma: a multi- institutional analysis of 434 patients. Arch Surg 2012;147(12):1107–1113

10. Kennedy AS, McNeillie P, Dezarn WA, et al. Treatment parameters and outcome in 680 treatments of internal radiation with resin ^{90}Y-microspheres for unresectable hepatic tumors. Int J Radiat Oncol Biol Phys 2009;74(5):1494–1500

11. Burke EC, Jarnagin WR, Hochwald SN, Pisters PW, Fong Y, Blumgart LH. Hilar cholangiocarcinoma: patterns of spread, the importance of hepatic resection for curative operation, and a presurgical clinical staging system. Ann Surg 1998;228(3):385–394

12. Jarnagin WR, Fong Y, DeMatteo RP, et al. Staging, resectability, and outcome in 225 patients with hilar cholangiocarcinoma. Ann Surg 2001;234(4):507–517, discussion 517–519

13. Darwish Murad S, Kim WR, Harnois DM, et al. Efficacy of neoadjuvant chemoradiation, followed by liver transplantation, for perihilar cholangiocarcinoma at 12 US centers. Gastroenterology 2012;143(1):88–98.e3, quiz e14

14. Hii MW, Gibson RN, Speer AG, Collier NA, Sherson N, Jardine C. Role of radiology in the treatment of malignant hilar biliary strictures 2: 10 years of single-institution experience with percutaneous treatment. Australas Radiol 2003;47(4):393–403

15. Cheng Q, Luo X, Zhang B, Jiang X, Yi B, Wu M. Distal bile duct carcinoma: prognostic factors after curative surgery. A series of 112 cases. Ann Surg Oncol 2007;14(3):1212–1219

16. Murakami Y, Uemura K, Hayashidani Y, Sudo T, Ohge H, Sueda T. Pancreatoduodenectomy for distal cholangiocarcinoma: prognostic impact of lymph node metastasis. World J Surg 2007;31(2):337–342, discussion 343–344

17. Randi G, Franceschi S, La Vecchia C. Gallbladder cancer worldwide: geographical distribution and risk factors. Int J Cancer 2006;118(7):1591–1602

18. Maringhini A, Moreau JA, Melton LJ III, Hench VS, Zinsmeister AR, DiMagno EP. Gallstones, gallbladder cancer, and other gastrointestinal malignancies. An epidemiologic study in Rochester, Minnesota. Ann Intern Med 1987;107(1):30–35

19. Chijiiwa K, Kimura H, Tanaka M. Malignant potential of the gallbladder in patients with anomalous pancreaticobiliary ductal junction. The difference in risk between patients with and without choledochal cyst. Int Surg 1995;80(1):61–64

20. Tokiwa K, Iwai N. Early mucosal changes of the gallbladder in patients with anomalous arrangement of the pancreaticobiliary duct. Gastroenterology 1996;110(5):1614–1618

21. Perpetuo MD, Valdivieso M, Heilbrun LK, Nelson RS, Connor T, Bodey GP. Natural history study of gallbladder cancer: a review of 36 years experience at M. D. Anderson Hospital and Tumor Institute. Cancer 1978;42(1):330–335

22. Albores-Saavedra J, Henson DE. Atlas of Tumor Pathology. 2nd ed. Fascicle 22: Tumors of the Gallbladder and Extrahepatic Bile Ducts. Washington, DC: Armed Forces Institute of Pathology; 1986

23. Hanada K, Itoh M, Fujii K, Tsuchida A, Ooishi H, Kajiyama G. K-ras and p53 mutations in stage I gallbladder carcinoma with an anomalous junction of the pancreaticobiliary duct. Cancer 1996;77(3):452–458

24. Uno T, Itami J, Aruga M, Araki H, Tani M, Kobori O. Primary carcinoma of the gallbladder: role of external beam radiation therapy in patients with locally advanced tumor. Strahlenther Onkol 1996;172(9):496–500

25. Todoroki T, Iwasaki Y, Orii K, et al. Resection combined with intraoperative radiation therapy (IORT) for stage IV (TNM) gallbladder carcinoma. World J Surg 1991;15(3):357–366

26. Eckel F, Brunner T, Jelic S; ESMO Guidelines Working Group. Biliary cancer: ESMO Clinical Practice Guidelines for diagnosis, treatment and follow-up. Ann Oncol 2011;22(Suppl 6):vi40–vi44

27. Kresl JJ, Schild SE, Henning GT, et al. Adjuvant external beam radiation therapy with concurrent chemotherapy in the management of gallbladder carcinoma. Int J Radiat Oncol Biol Phys 2002;52(1):167–175

28. Mäkelä JT, Kairaluoma MI. Superselective intra-arterial chemotherapy with mitomycin for gallbladder cancer. Br J Surg 1993;80(7):912–915

11   Lung Cancer (Non–Small Cell)

Douglas M. Coldwell

Epidemiology

Lung cancer is the most common cause of cancer death worldwide. It is associated with smoking, but over half the cases in the United States are diagnosed in patients who never smoked or quit many years earlier. Also, asbestos, beryllium, cadmium, chromium, radon gas, nickel, and vinyl chloride, which the patients are exposed to at the workplace and in the environment, are causative agents.[1–3]

Pathology

Adenocarcinoma is the dominant type, followed by squamous cell.

Genetics

Carcinogens in smoking are responsible for deoxyribonucleic acid (DNA) adduct formation and DNA mutations that activate the v-Ki-ras2 Kirsten rat sarcoma viral oncogene homolog (*KRAS*) oncogene seen in 25% of patients.[4,5] Nonsquamous mutations include epidermal growth factor receptor (*EGFR*), anaplastic lymphoma kinase (*ALK*) rearrangement, *ROS1* rearrangement, human epidermal growth factor receptor 2 (*HER2*) mutation, v-Raf murine sarcoma viral oncogene homolog B (*BRAF*) mutation, rearranged during transfection (*RET*) rearrangement, *KRAS*, mesenchymal–epithelial transition (*MET*) mutation, *MEK1* mutation, *PIK3CA* mutation. This plethora of gene mutations has led to the development of targeted agents. The first four mutations have agents that have been approved by the Food and Drug Administration (FDA). These include gefitinib (*EGFR* inhibitor), erlotinib (*EGFR* inhibitor), afatinib (*EGFR* inhibitor, *HER2* inhibitor), crizotinib (*ALK* inhibitor, *ROS1* inhibitor), and ceritinib (*ALK* inhibitor).[6] Multiple companies are now providing gene sequencing services to detect the mutations that can have drugs targeted to them. Practically, for the interventional radiology, this requires a larger biopsy specimen, usually cores, which will increase the likelihood of a pneumothorax in an already at-risk population due to chronic obstructive pulmonary disease or emphysema caused by smoking.

Staging[7]

Tumor

- T1a = Primary tumor is 2 cm or less in diameter.
- T1b = Primary tumor is greater than 2 but less than 3 cm in diameter.
- T2a = Primary tumor is greater than 3 but less than 5 cm in diameter.
- T2b = Primary tumor is greater than 5 but less than 7 cm in diameter.
- T3 = Primary tumor is greater than 7 cm in diameter.
- T3 invasive = Invades chest wall, diaphragm, phrenic nerve, mediastinal pleura, or pericardium.
- T3 central = Primary tumor is less than 2 cm to the carina or atelectasis of an entire lung.
- T3 satellite = Any size primary tumor with additional tumor nodules in the same ipsilateral lobe.
- T4 invasive = Any size tumor that invades heart, great vessels, esophagus, trachea, vertebral body, carina.
- T4 ipsilateral nodules = Separate tumor nodule in a different ipsilateral lobe.

Lymph Nodes

The lymph nodes in the chest are divided into levels so that communication about positive nodal spread can be uniform.

- Level 1 = Highest mediastinal nodes at the upper rim of the brachiocephalic vein where it crosses anteriorly to the trachea.
- Level 2 = Upper paratracheal nodes.
- Level 3 = Prevascular and retrotracheal nodes.
- Level 4 = Lower paratracheal nodes.
- Level 5 = Aortopulmonary window nodes.
- Level 6 = Para-aortic nodes near the ascending aorta or phrenic nerve.
- Level 7 = Subcarinal nodes.
- Level 8 = Paraesophageal nodes below the carina.
- Level 9 = Pulmonary ligament nodes.
- Level 10 = Hilar nodes.
- Level 11 = Interlobar nodes.
- Level 12 = Lobar nodes.
- Level 13 = Segmental nodes.
- Level 14 = Subsegmental nodes.

These levels are preceded by an R or L designating the side, as in R10 node.[8]

The staging for nodal extension is as follows:

- N0 = No nodal metastases.
- N1 = Nodal metastases in ipsilateral hilar, peribronchial, or pulmonary nodes.
- N2 = Nodal metastases in ipsilateral mediastinal or subcarinal nodes.
- N3 = Metastases in contralateral nodes.

Metastases

- M0 = No distant metastases.
- M1 = Metastases in contralateral lobe, pleural nodules, or malignant pleural effusion.
- M2 = Distant metastases.

Stages

- Stage 0 = Carcinoma in situ.
- Stage I = T1a/b, T2a; N0, M0.
- Stage IIA = T1, T2a; N1, M0 or T2b, N0, M0.
- Stage IIB = T2b, N1, M0 or T3, N0, M0.
- Stage IIIA = T1, T2, T3; N2, M0 or T3, T4; N1, M0 or T4, N0 or N1, M0.
- Stage IIIB = Any T, N3, M0 or T4, N2, M0.
- Stage IVA = Any T, Any N, M1.
- Stage IVB = Any T, Any N, M2.

If there are no distant metastases, it becomes crucial to know the status of the mediastinal lymph nodes. A fluorodeoxyglucose positron emission tomography (FDG-PET)/computed tomography (CT) scan will demonstrate any node greater than 1 cm in diameter is likely involved with tumor. However, nodes that are suspicious on CT need to be biopsied via either bronchoscopy or mediastinoscopy.

Treatment

Surgery

Minimally invasive resection using video-assisted thoracic surgery (VATS) has dramatically decreased the morbidity of lung cancer surgery, allowing more fragile patients to have the tumor excised.

The treatment of non–small cell lung cancer (NSCLC) requires a combination of surgery, chemotherapy, and radiation that is personalized for each patient considering their comorbidities and the stage of the disease. The recommended treatments for each stage are as follows:

- Stage I: A minimally invasive, for example, VATS, lobectomy is recommended without adjuvant chemotherapy or radiation for patients who can tolerate the surgery with a 5-year survival of 60 to 80%. In compromised patients, the use of Stereotactic Body Radiation Therapy (SBRT) can be substituted for surgery with a 2-year survival of 60 and 45% at 5 years. Disease control at the primary site is accomplished with SBRT in 80 to 100% at 2 years.
- Stage II: Resection followed by adjuvant chemotherapy is the standard of care, with survival at 5 years of 45%, and most deaths (75%) are caused by recurrence. The chemotherapy recommended is a doublet that includes cisplatin. Often used for the other half of the doublet are vinorelbine or etoposide. In locally invasive T3N0M0 tumors, an en bloc resection is recommended. If all the tumor is removed, a 50 to 60% 5-year survival is expected. If less than an R0 resection is performed, the survival is less than 5% at 5 years, with or without radiotherapy. For central T3N0 tumors, even with R0 resection the survival is 25 to 30% at 5 years.[8,9]
  Pancoast tumors are a subset of T3 tumors. These occur at the apex of the lung and invade the thoracic inlet effecting the first rib, brachial plexus, subclavian artery and vein, and thoracic spine. Neoadjuvant chemoradiation utilizing a cisplatin doublet and at least 45 Gy of external beam radiation therapy (EBRT) is recommended. Surgery is performed for cure and, if an R0 resection is performed, 5-year survival is approximately 55% with a recurrence rate of 6%. However, if such a resection cannot be accomplished, chemoradiation should be performed for cure with a 5-year survival of 28%.[10,11]
- Stage III is conveniently subdivided into three clinical subgroups:
  - Where there is unsuspected N2 disease prior to surgery. Adjuvant chemotherapy with a cisplatin doublet extended overall survival (OS) to 20% at 5 years. When radiation is added postoperatively, the OS rises to 27 to 33%. If combined with

cisplatin doublet, chemoradiation has a higher toxicity than when given sequentially. Adjuvant radiation should be considered if an incomplete resection is performed. If an R0 resection is performed, no adjuvant therapy is recommended.[12,13]

– Where there is discrete nodal involvement detected on CT or PET/CT prior to surgery. Mediastinoscopy with nodal sampling should be performed at the time of initial surgery. Meta-analyses of intent to treat studies have suggested that the outcomes are better after neoadjuvant chemotherapy.[9,14] Several randomized clinical trials compared neoadjuvant therapy followed by surgery to chemotherapy alone and found no significant difference.[14] Chemoradiotherapy using a cisplatin doublet with 45 Gy of EBRT concurrently resulted in better outcomes than chemotherapy alone with higher rates of mediastinal downstaging, higher rates of near pathologic complete response, and lower rates of incomplete resection.[9,14]

– Where there is infiltrative tumor or matted lymph nodes defined in CT or PET/CT. Radiation alone has been the historical modality used to control the tumor in this case with an OS of 22% at 5 years.[15] With the advent of combined modality therapy, chemoradiation is recommended with a cisplatin doublet. Using this therapy, there is a 30% reduction in mortality at 2 years when compared with radiation alone.[16] Use of cisplatin and pemetrexed disodium offers a lower toxicity profile than cisplatin and etoposide with 63 Gy of EBRT, but there is no improvement in survival with OS of 25 months.[17]

• Stage IV: Patients with this level of advanced disease are often symptomatic and are more concerned with quality of life than undergoing toxic chemotherapy. However, it has been shown that patients live longer with the administration of chemotherapy than by the use of best supportive care, and the toxicity of this chemotherapy is less than grade III.[18] It is recommended that patients with stage IV NSCLC be treated with chemotherapy with a platinum doublet avoiding pemetrexed, if squamous, then maintain with erlotinib. If nonsquamous, the patients should have genetic testing to determine if a genetic alteration conforming to the requirements of a specific targeted drug is present. If the mutation is present, treat with the specific drug. If not, treat with a platinum doublet and bevacizumab if possible. Then maintain with bevacizumab (if eligible), erlotinib, or pemetrexed.[9] If patients are treated with targeted therapy, their survival ranges from 20 to 36 months with an overall response rate of 25 to 74%. The use of maintenance chemotherapy extends the survival from 10 to 12 months.[19]

Chemotherapy

Most chemotherapy regimens are based on cisplatin plus another agent, usually vinorelbine, etoposide, or pemetrexed. When specific genetic mutations are noted, agents such as crizotinib are utilized primarily in younger nonsmoking patients with *ALK* fusion mutation who do not have *EGFR* or *KRAS* mutations. Unfortunately, these genetic targetable mutations are only a few percent of the patients, but when found they may show a dramatic response.

Role of Interventional Radiology

In the diagnosis of lung cancer, CT or fluoroscopically guided biopsies are common. It is imperative that a cytopathologist be present for these procedures to determine if diagnostic tissue is obtained. This will result in more successful biopsies with fewer "nondiagnostic" reports. The use of genetic targeting has required an increase in the number of cells obtained. Many institutions are using only core specimens to insure that the cell yield is high. This does, however, as mentioned earlier, increase the rate of pneumothorax from the current 30% to likely 50 to 60% and a higher rate of chest tube placements. The informed consent for the biopsy should also include a provision for placement of a chest tube since the patient will be sedated and not able to sign for it later when time may be short.

Solitary lesions or a small number of lesions can also be treated with radiofrequency or microwave ablation with very good success. Lesions 3 cm and smaller can reliably be treated without the side effects of radiation. Since the ablation probes are approximately 14 gauge, it is almost assured that the patient will need a chest tube. These tubes need to remain in place for at least 24 hours so that the pleural injury can heal; otherwise, a bronchopleural fistula may occur.

Hemoptysis is a common problem in patients with lung cancer. This can be treated with bronchoscopy-directed laser/cauterization, radiation, or bronchial artery embolization. If the latter is chosen, care must be taken to perform careful angiography to determine if the anterior spinal artery is present. It usually arises from the right and has a characteristic "hairpin" shape. If it is found, the embolization should be distal to its origin via a microcatheter insuring that no reflux of particles occurs. Particles no smaller than 100 μ should be used and liquid embolics must be avoided. If the anterior spinal artery is embolized, a transverse myelitis will occur with near immediate bilateral lower extremity paralysis. This paralysis may resolve with time and rehabilitation. The formation of collateral arteries to the anterior spinal artery or reticular arteries may be caused by irradiation of the tumor and the surrounding lung. The hemoptysis is very likely to be stopped by the embolization of the bronchial artery. If the arteries to the tumor are completely occluded, the bleeding may halt and the tumor may necrose. The patient should be forewarned that they may cough up small pieces of necrotic tumor.

Encroachment of a lung tumor onto the superior vena cava (SVC) may result in the near occlusion of the SVC and causing the SVC syndrome of cyanosis, plethora, edema of the upper body, enlarged superficial veins, dyspnea, and cough. Rarely, cerebral edema and laryngeal stridor may occur. The acuity of the onset is directly related to the severity of the symptoms. A tumor that slowly occludes the SVC allows collateral veins to open into the azygous system and the patient may not show any of the symptoms. However, when the SVC syndrome is present, it is a straightforward procedure to access the right internal jugular vein and place a catheter through an 11-Fr sheath into the SVC and cross the stenosis. As soon as the lesion is dilated so that the initial stent can be placed, the patient always states that they can feel the pressure in their upper body release. A 12- to 16-mm-diameter stent should then be placed across the lesion, insuring that there is at least 1 cm of stent beyond the stenosis on either side. The stents may be balloon expandable, but the pain caused to the patient is excruciating. Many prefer to use self-expanding stents so that a 12-mm diameter can be dilated to 10 mm and open to its maximal diameter slowly.

Chronic malignant pleural effusions are often present in lung cancer patients. These can be managed with serial thoracenteses, but if the time between them is a week or 10 days, that is an indication for the placement of a tunneled chest tube. This catheter is 16 Fr, multiside holed and made from polyurethane so that it is soft and well tolerated. A tunnel is anesthetized along the lateral wall of the chest and the catheter placed through it, similar to the placement of a dialysis or Hickman catheter. The pleural space is punctured under ultrasound guidance and a peel-away sheath is placed. The catheter is then placed into the pleural cavity. Vacuum bottles are arranged to be delivered to the patient and they may drain their effusions at home, saving them a trip to the hospital. It should be noted that there needs to be a significant pleural effusion present so that the tube may be positioned without any damage to the lung.

Pain is one of the hallmarks of lung cancer and its metastases. Erosion into the chest wall may be initially treated with radiation, but it takes several weeks for this therapy to take effect. It is an option to ablate the intercostal nerves that supply the area of chest wall erosion and immediately the pain will decrease or vanish. Use of a 25-gauge needle is usually sufficient to inject the nerves at least 10 cm from the spinous process with ethanol having anesthetized the nerve with lidocaine immediately before. Approximately 5 to 10 mL of ethanol is used for each intercostal nerve. If pain is elicited, administer more lidocaine, then continue. Longer acting anesthetics are not necessary as the pain is short-lived and these require time to take effect, while lidocaine's time to cause anesthesia is essentially immediate.

Pain due to bony metastases is also a huge problem with lung cancer patients. The cancer may metastasize to the spine causing vertebral compression fractures (VCF) and spinal cord compression. If magnetic resonance imaging demonstrates that such a VCF is present, augmentation is indicated. Since there is tumor present in the spine, even though the patient may have already had radiotherapy, the vertebral body should be ablated with radiofrequency ablation (RFA), then filled with polymethyl methacrylate cement, which will also heat the tumor and cause more tumor death, but it will prevent the fracture fragments from moving against each other, which is a cause of the pain. Performing RFA on the tumor initially allows the formation of a void that is then filled with cement and ideally will intercalate between the trabeculae to reinforce the bone. Height of the vertebral body may or may not increase, but given the tumor presence, it makes little difference to the pain alleviation. This is successful in approximately 85% of patients.[20] If the posterior wall of the vertebral body is eroded by tumor, the polymethyl methacrylate (PMMA) cement may flow into the spinal canal, causing more pain and an immediate operation to remove the cement. It has been shown that a thick cement can be placed across the transverse aspect of the vertebral body to act as a dam keeping the remainder of the cement anterior to it. This is only possible if an osteotome is placed through the access bone biopsy needle cutting a channel across the vertebral body for the cement to follow.[21] This RFA followed by PMMA cement placement is applicable to almost any site where the tumor may metastasize.[22]

References

1. Tong L, Spitz MR, Fueger JJ, Amos CA. Lung carcinoma in former smokers. Cancer 1996;78(5):1004–1010

2. Garces YI, Yang P, Parkinson J, et al. The relationship between cigarette smoking and quality of life after lung cancer diagnosis. Chest 2004;126(6):1733–1741

3. Visbal AL, Williams BA, Nichols FC III, et al. Gender differences in non-small-cell lung cancer survival: an analysis of 4,618 patients diagnosed between 1997 and 2002. Ann Thorac Surg 2004;78(1):209–215, discussion 215

4. Hoffmann D, Djordjevic MV, Rivenson A, Zang E, Desai D, Amin S. A study of tobacco carcinogenesis. LI. Relative potencies of tobacco-specific N-nitrosamines as inducers of lung tumours in A/J mice. Cancer Lett 1993;71(1-3):25–30

5. Belinsky SA, Devereux TR, Maronpot RR, Stoner GD, Anderson MW. Relationship between the formation of promutagenic adducts and the activation of the K-ras protooncogene in lung tumors from A/J mice treated with nitrosamines. Cancer Res 1989;49(19):5305–5311

6. Imielinski M, Berger AH, Hammerman PS, et al. Mapping the hallmarks of lung adenocarcinoma with massively parallel sequencing. Cell 2012;150(6):1107–1120

7. Detterbeck FC, Boffa DJ, Tanoue LT. The new lung cancer staging system. Chest 2009;136(1):260–271

8. Mountain CF, Dresler CM. Regional lymph node classification for lung cancer staging. Chest 1997;111(6):1718–1723

9. Howington JA, Blum MG, Chang AC, Balekian AA, Murthy SC. Treatment of stage I and II non-small cell lung cancer: diagnosis and management of lung cancer, 3rd ed: American College of Chest Physicians evidence-based clinical practice guidelines. Chest 2013; 143(5, Suppl):e278S–e313S

10. National Comprehensive Cancer Network. Clinical Practice Guidelines in Oncology. Non-Small Cell Lung Cancer, Version 6. 2017. Fort Washington, PA: National Comprehensive Cancer Network; 2017

11. Kozower BD, Larner JM, Detterbeck FC, Jones DR. Special treatment issues in non-small cell lung cancer: Diagnosis and management of lung cancer, 3rd ed: American College of Chest Physicians evidence-based clinical practice guidelines. Chest 2013; 143(5, Suppl):e369S–e399S

12. Foroulis CN, Zarogoulidis P, Darwiche K, et al. Superior sulcus (Pancoast) tumors: current evidence on diagnosis and radical treatment. J Thorac Dis 2013;5(Suppl 4):S342–S358

13. Detterbeck F. What to do with "Surprise" N2?: intraoperative management of patients with non-small cell lung cancer. J Thorac Oncol 2008;3(3):289–302

14. Keller SM, Adak S, Wagner H, et al; Eastern Cooperative Oncology Group. A randomized trial of postoperative adjuvant therapy in patients with completely resected stage II or IIIA non-small-cell lung cancer. N Engl J Med 2000;343(17):1217–1222

15. Ramnath N, Dilling TJ, Harris LJ, et al. Treatment of stage III non-small cell lung cancer: Diagnosis and management of lung cancer, 3rd ed: American College of Chest Physicians evidence-based clinical practice guidelines. Chest 2013; 143(5, Suppl)e314S–e340S

16. Perez CA, Stanley K, Rubin P, et al. A prospective randomized study of various irradiation doses and fractionation schedules in the treatment of inoperable non-oat-cell carcinoma of the lung. Preliminary report by the Radiation Therapy Oncology Group. Cancer 1980;45(11):2744–2753

17. Marino P, Preatoni A, Cantoni A. Randomized trials of radiotherapy alone versus combined chemotherapy and radiotherapy in stages IIIa and IIIb nonsmall cell lung cancer. A meta-analysis. Cancer 1995;76(4):593–601

18. Senan S, Brade A, Wang LH, et al. PROCLAIM: randomized phase III trial of pemetrexed-cisplatin or etoposide-cisplatin plus thoracic radiation therapy followed by consolidation chemotherapy in locally advanced nonsquamous non-small-cell lung cancer. J Clin Oncol 2016;34(9):953–962

19. Socinski MA, Evans T, Gettinger S, et al. Treatment of stage IV non-small cell lung cancer: Diagnosis and management of lung cancer, 3rd ed: American College of Chest Physicians evidence-based clinical practice guidelines. Chest 2013; 143(5, Suppl)e341S–e368S

20. Paz-Ares LG, de Marinis F, Dediu M, et al. PARAMOUNT: final overall survival results of the phase III study of maintenance pemetrexed versus placebo immediately after induction treatment with pemetrexed plus cisplatin for advanced nonsquamous non-small-cell lung cancer. J Clin Oncol 2013;31(23):2895–2902

21. Anchala PR, Irving WD, Hillen TJ, et al. Treatment of metastatic spinal lesions with a navigational bipolar radiofrequency ablation device: a multicenter retrospective study. Pain Physician 2014;17(4):317–327

22. Hirsch AE, Jha RM, Yoo AJ, et al. The use of vertebral augmentation and external beam radiation therapy in the multimodal management of malignant vertebral compression fractures. Pain Physician 2011;14(5):447–458

12 Head and Neck Cancer

Douglas M. Coldwell

Epidemiology

Head and neck cancer is usually associated with alcohol and tobacco use.[1]

Pathology

Usually squamous cell carcinoma that, if small, will spread to ipsilateral nodes, but if abuts midline or is large, it may spread to contralateral nodes.[2]

Genetics

Human papilloma virus (HPV) infection also plays a role and those tumors related to HPV have a better prognosis since these patients present younger and are less likely to have a significant alcohol and tobacco history. They do, however, have a history of multiple sex partners and are less likely to have a second primary tumor.[3]

Staging[4]

Tumor

- T1 = 2 cm or less in diameter.
- T2 = 2 to 4 cm in diameter.
- T3 = Greater than 4 cm in diameter.
- T4 = Tumors that invade or encase adjacent structures.

Lymph Nodes

Lymph nodes are classified by levels:

- I = Submental and submandibular.
- II = Superior third of jugular vein nodes, from digastric muscle to carotid bifurcation.
- III = Middle third of jugular vein nodes, from carotid bifurcation to cricothyroid notch or omohyoid muscle.
- IV = Lower third of jugular vein nodes, from cricothyroid notch or omohyoid muscle to the clavicle.
- V = Posterior triangle nodes and supraclavicular nodes.
- VI = Anterior compartment nodes from hyoid bone to suprasternal notch.
- N1 = Metastasis in a single ipsilateral node that is 3 cm or less in greatest dimension.
- N2a = Single ipsilateral node is 3 to 6 cm in greatest dimension.
- N2b = Metastasis in multiple ipsilateral nodes is not greater than 6 cm in greatest dimension.
- N2c = Metastasis in bilateral or contralateral nodes is not greater than 6 cm in greatest dimension.
- N3 = Metastasis in node is great than 6 cm in greatest dimension.

Metastases

- M0 = No metastases.
- M1 = Metastases present.

Staging

- Stage I = T1N0M0.
- Stage II = T2N0M0.
- Stage III = T3N0M0 or T1–T3N1M0.
- Stage IVA = T4a, N0–1, M0.
- Stage IVB = Any T, N3M0 or T4b, any N, M0.
- Stage IVC = Any T, any N, M1.

Treatment

Surgery

Resection of the tumor is a mainstay of therapy for this tumor. A neck dissection is performed to evaluate the lymph nodes in levels I to V. The radical neck dissection will remove all nodes and the contiguous structures including the sternocleidomastoid muscle, the omohyoid muscle, internal and external jugular veins, cranial nerve XI, and the submandibular gland. The modified radical neck dissection will spare cranial nerve XI (type I), cranial nerve XI and the internal jugular vein (type 2), or cranial nerve XI, the internal jugular vein, and the sternocleidomastoid muscle (type3). The last is considered to be the most functional result.[5]

Patients are considered to be at low risk (20%) for neck disease when it is not clinically evident in T1 tumors of the floor of mouth, oral tongue, retromolar trigone, gingiva, hard palate, or buccal mucosa (group 1). Those at intermediate risk (20–30%) include those patients with T1 tumors of the soft palate, pharyngeal wall, supraglottic larynx, or tonsil or T2 tumors of group 1 mentioned earlier. Those patients at high (>30%) risk of neck disease are those with T1–T4 tumors of the nasopharynx, pyriform sinus, base of tongue or T2–T4 tumors or the soft palate pharyngeal wall, supraglottic larynx, or tonsil, or T3–T4 tumors of the earlier-mentioned group 1. Patients who develop lymph node metastases in the neck after having the primary tumor successfully addressed by surgery or radiotherapy (RT) have a salvage rate of 50 to 60%.[6] An elective neck dissection is indicated when the risk of nodal spread is 10 to 15%. Modified neck dissection techniques can be used with better functional results. Patients found to have nodal disease are then treated with RT or chemoradiotherapy.

The surgery for these lesions is obviously complex and requires the use of free flaps transposed to cover the defects. Transoral robotic surgery (TORS) is the latest minimally invasive technique to be utilized to treat lesions in the oral cavity.[7]

Chemotherapy

Those tumors that have invaded adjacent structures or have nodal metastases or distant metastases are candidates for management primarily or neoadjuvantly with chemoradiotherapy. This is an external beam radiation therapy (EBRT) given up to 70 to 100 Gy combined with continuous infusion 5-FU given as a radiation sensitizer. About 80 to 90% of oropharyngeal tumors are HPV positive. And most of these are sensitive to the combination of concurrent carboplatin and taxol with radiation.[8]

Cisplatin is the foundation of modern chemotherapy for these tumors. It is commonly given at 75 to 100 mg/m^2 every 3 to 4 weeks. The usual side effects from cisplatin are seen: renal failure, peripheral neuropathies, ototoxicity (tinnitus), and gastrointestinal (nausea and vomiting) toxicity. These are usually able to be managed symptomatically. The survival with cisplatin is approximately 5 to 6 months. Single agent taxane (either paclitaxel or docetaxel) or methotrexate has also been used. In patients who are refractory to cisplatin and express epidermal growth factor receptor (EGFR), cetuximab is used. Combination therapy with 5-FU and cisplatin achieves a 50 to 70% response rate and a 16 to 27% complete response rate with survival in recurrent or metastatic head and neck cancer of 5 to 6 months.[9–11] The combination of intense chemotherapy with radiation therapy with potential surgery leaves the patients nutritionally depleted and unable to swallow due to mucositis. A percutaneous gastrostomy is usually placed for feeding.[12]

Radiotherapy

Usually external beam radiation therapy to 70 to 100 Gy is used in combination with chemotherapy as a sensitizer. Occasionally, high dose rate brachytherapy seeds have been used and implanted during surgery to treat questionable remaining tumor. Recurrences in the maximally irradiated bed of the tumor are extremely difficult to manage since additional radiation may result in necrosis of tissues, and systemic chemotherapies are limited in effectiveness to recurrent tumor.[11] Usually cisplatin is combined with cetuximab with a 20 to 30% response rate and a median survival of 4 to 6 m.[10] Unfortunately, when the tumor recurs, it is often with excruciating pain that is very difficult to manage with oral or intravenous opiates. A small pilot study carried out using superselective intra-arterial (IA) infusion of cisplatin (75 mg/m^2) over 20 minutes given every 2 weeks for an average of two infusions into the most distal position where the catheter has coverage of the entire tumor. Complete response was seen in 4/12 patients (33%), partial response in 3/12 (25%), and stabilization of disease in 3/12 (25%) for a disease stabilization rate of 83%. Symptoms were eliminated in 10/12 patients (83%).[13]

Locoregional

Given the use of transarterial infusion of chemotherapy in other sites, the possibility of use of IA cisplatin into the external carotid artery with radiation immediately following was investigated and found to be of no assistance in extending the overall survival (OS) or the response rate.[8] However, in patients who have recurrent or resistant disease, the use of IA cisplatin as described earlier has an impressive response.

In patients with tonsillar cancer especially, the risk of carotid blowout syndrome occurring is higher than usual. The risk is related to the fact that all these patients have had surgery, a flap placed, and maximal radiation to the area. Patients will present with gross hematemesis and will die quickly if they are not transported to the interventional radiology (IR) suite immediately where a covered vascular stent can be place in the common carotid artery that may extend to the internal carotid artery. If the external carotid artery is bypassed, it should be coil embolized to prevent the back bleeding due to the cross-collateralization in the neck. The risk of carotid blowout syndrome is related to the amount of the periphery of the carotid artery that is surrounded by tumor. If more than half of the circumference is surrounded by tumor, the risk is significant.

Head and neck tumors may erode into adjacent arteries and cause bleeding that is serious but not explosive carotid blowout syndrome. Usually the internal maxillary artery is involved. Due to the collaterals to the ophthalmic artery and to the brain, small particles or glue should not be used; only coils should be used.

When carotid body tumors or glomus jugulare tumors are present, they may be embolized to facilitate surgery or to palliate the patient. These tumors usually have a single artery supplying them, a branch of the ascending pharyngeal artery. Care must be taken in this artery as it has branches that feed the base of the skull and anastomose with the anterior and posterior cerebral circulation. Use of smaller microcatheters and early polymerizing NBCA (*n*-Butyl cyanoacrylate) glue or 100-µ-diameter particles are recommended. These tumors are highly vascular and may shunt to form an almost arteriovenous malformation appearance with tortuous venous outflow.

Additional support IR can give to these patients is the placement of both subcutaneous ports and percutaneous gastrostomies. These are normally placed simultaneously early in their treatment.

Prognosis

Surgery and RT are the only means of cure for head and neck cancer. Chemotherapy will enhance the effects of RT and is commonly used in patients with stage III or IV disease. Most centers will start with surgery in those patients who are candidates and save RT for recurrence or an R1 or R2 resection. Cisplatin-based chemoradiotherapy has a higher rate of progression-free survival (60–70%) as well as OS (70–80%) when compared with RT alone. In general, T1 lesions have about an 80% overall 5-year survival, T2 a 70% OS, T3 a 50% OS, and T4 a 15% OS.

References

1. Blot WJ, McLaughlin JK, Winn DM, et al. Smoking and drinking in relation to oral and pharyngeal cancer. Cancer Res 1988;48(11):3282–3287

2. Fisch U. Lymphography of the Cervical Lymphatic System. Philadelphia, PA: W. B. Saunders; 1968

3. Ang KK, Harris J, Wheeler R, et al. Human papillomavirus and survival of patients with oropharyngeal cancer. N Engl J Med 2010;363(1):24–35

4. Edge SB, Byrd DR, Compton CC. AJCC Cancer Staging Manual. Vol 7. New York, NY: Springer; 2010

5. DaVita VT, Lawrence TS, Rosenberg SA. Cancer: Principles and Practice of Oncology, 10th ed. Philadelphia, PA: Wolters, Kluwer; 2015

6. Mendenhall WM, Million RR. Elective neck irradiation for squamous cell carcinoma of the head and neck: analysis of time-dose factors and causes of failure. Int J Radiat Oncol Biol Phys 1986;12(5):741–746

7. Loevner LA, Learned KO, Mohan S, et al. Transoral robotic surgery in head and neck cancer: what radiologists need to know about the cutting edge. Radiographics 2013;33(6):1759–1779

8. Mallen-St Clair J, Alani M, Wang MB, Srivatsan ES. Human papillomavirus in oropharyngeal cancer: The changing face of a disease. Biochim Biophys Acta 2016;1866(2):141–150

9. Herbst RS, Arquette M, Shin DM, et al. Phase II multicenter study of the epidermal growth factor receptor antibody cetuximab and cisplatin for recurrent and refractory squamous cell carcinoma of the head and neck. J Clin Oncol 2005;23(24):5578–5587

10. Trigo J, Hitt R, Koralweski P, et al. Cetuximab monotherapy is active in patients (pts) with platinum-refractory recurrent/metastatic squamous cell carcinoma of the head and neck (SCCHN): Results of a phase II study. J Clin Oncol 2004;22:S5502

11. Burtness B, Goldwasser MA, Flood W, Mattar B, Forastiere AA; Eastern Cooperative Oncology Group. Phase III randomized trial of cisplatin plus placebo compared with cisplatin plus cetuximab in metastatic/recurrent head and neck cancer: an Eastern Cooperative Oncology Group study. J Clin Oncol 2005;23(34):8646–8654

12. Bishop S, Reed WM. The provision of enteral nutritional support during definitive chemoradiotherapy in head and neck cancer patients. J Med Radiat Sci 2015;62(4):267–276

13. Coldwell DM, VanEcho DD, Murthy R, Boyd-Kranis RL, Hastings GS, Radack DM. Treatment ofradioresistant head and neck squamous cell carcinomas (HNSCC) with superselective intra-arterial infusion of platinol. SCVIR Annual Meeting, March 2001

13   Renal Cell Carcinoma

Douglas M. Coldwell

Epidemiology

Incidence of renal cell carcinoma (RCC) has been increasing by 2 to 3% per decade. It is usually found in the developed world. Incidence in Asians is low; it is highest in the United States in African Americans. It is found mostly in patients over 65 years old. Risk factors include smoking, obesity, hypertension and occupational exposure to asbestos, lead, cadmium, petrochemicals.[1–3]

Pathology

RCC is derived from the nephron.

There are three major histologic types of RCC:

- Clear cell RCC: Derived from proximal tubules, 60 to 70% of cases, sporadic and not linked to syndromes.
- Papillary RCC: Derived from proximal tubules, 10 to 15% of cases, less aggressive than clear cell RCC, may be hereditary.
- Chromophobe RCC: Derived from cortical collecting duct, 3 to 5% of cases, least aggressive RCC, sporadic but may be associated with Birt–Hogg–Dubé syndrome.

Birt–Hogg–Dubé syndrome: autosomal-dominant mutation in Folliculin (*FLCN*) gene (*17p11*), multiple chromophobe RCC, oncocytomas, renal and pulmonary cysts, fibrofolliculomas, spontaneous pneumothorax.[4,5]

Rare types of RCC include the following:

- Multilocular cystic: Favorable prognosis after removal.
- Carcinoma of the collecting ducts of Bellini: Very rare, high-grade, poor prognosis, one-third with metastases at diagnosis, two-thirds die within 2 years.
- Medullary carcinoma: Very rare, almost all in patients with sickle cell disease or trait, very aggressive, 95% present with metastases, survival of 6 months.[6]

Genetics

- Clear cell RCC: Alteration of *chromosome 3p* in 70 to 90% with inactivation of von Hippel–Lindau gene by mutation and promoter hypermethylation. Multiple genetic mutations.[7–9]
- Papillary RCC: Trisomy or tetrasomy of *chromosome 17,* loss of *Y chromosome* in men.[10]Chromophobe RCC: Autosomal-dominant mutation in *FLCN* gene[11]
- Von Hippel–Lindau: Autosomal-dominant mutation in tumor suppressor gene *VHL* on *chromosome 3p25–3p26.* Associated are angiomatosis (usually in retina), central nervous system (CNS) or spinal hemangioblastoma, pheochromocytoma, clear cell RCC, pancreatic cysts. Usually multiple small clear cell or papillary RCC.[12]
- Tuberous sclerosis: Mutation in tuberous sclerosis 1 (*TSC1*) or tuberous sclerosis 2 (*TSC2*), which produces hamartin or tuberin, which are tumor suppressors. Associated with hamartomas (especially in CNS where they may be astrocytomas), multiple angiomyolipomas in kidney, polycystic kidney disease, rare clear cell RCC, dermal fibromas, and retinal phakomas, pulmonary lymphangiomyomatosis.[13,14]
- Cowden's syndrome: Mutation to *PTEN* (phosphatase and tensin homolog) gene (*10q23*). Associated with breast tumors, either benign or malignant, thyroid carcinoma, papillary RCC.[15]

Familial leiomyomatosis and RCC: Mutation in fumarate hydratase (*1q42–1q43*). Associated with papillary RCC, collecting duct RCC, leiomyomas of skin or uterus.

- Hereditary papillary RCC: Mutation in c-met proto-oncogene (*7q31*). Associated with multiple bilateral papillary RCC.[16]

Staging[17]

Tumor

- T1a = Less than 4 cm and confined to kidney.
- T1b = Greater than 4 cm but less than 7 cm and confined to kidney.
- T2a = Greater than 7 cm but less than 10 cm and confined to kidney.
- T2b = Greater than 10 cm and confined to kidney.
- T3a = Extension into renal vein or invades perirenal fat but not outside of **Gerota's fascia**.
- T3b = Extends into inferior vena cava below diaphragm.

- T3c = Extends into vena cava/right atrium above diaphragm or invades caval wall.
- T4 = Tumor invades beyond Gerota's fascia or into ipsilateral adrenal gland.

Lymph Nodes

- N0 = No regional lymph node metastases.
- N1 = Metastasis in regional lymph nodes.

Metastases

- M0 = No distant metastasis.
- M1 = Distant metastasis.
- Stage I = T1 N0 M0.
- Stage II = T2 N0 M0.
- Stage III = T3 Any N M0 or T1/T2 N1 M0.
- Stage IV = T4 Any N M0 or Any T, Any N, M1.

Treatment

Surgery

If it is T1/stage I, partial nephrectomy is performed with 1 to 2% recurrence. If tumor is less than and equal to 3 cm, radiofrequency ablation (RFA) or cryotherapy can be utilized with a slightly higher recurrence rate (5–8%) and similar prognosis. Contraindication to RFA is extension of the tumor into the collecting system.[18,19]

If it is T2/stage II, partial nephrectomy is the treatment of choice, if possible, but radical nephrectomy is usually performed. Evaluation of the lymph nodes is essential to determine if the stage is higher.[20,21]

If it is stage III or IV, the tumor is in an advanced stage with nodal or distant metastases. A cytoreductive nephrectomy can be performed and has been noted to be of both palliative and prognostic advantages.

Chemotherapy

Chemotherapy is usually utilized in metastatic RCC. The most common regimen is the use of high-dose interleukin-2 (IL-2) resulting in a sustained response for 5 to 7% of patients.[22] This therapy has been in use for over 20 years. Newer agents are targeted to immunological pathways. Nivolumab, which binds to the programmed death receptor-1 (PDR1), has shown a 30% overall response rate.[23] Since RCC is so hypervascular, a natural target would also be the vascular endothelial growth factor (VEGF) addressed by sunitinib, which also has activity against several tyrosine kinase receptors. RCC responds to sunitinib in 30 to 47% with a progression-free survival of 8.5 to 11 months and overall survival of 30 months.[24] Bevacizumab has also been utilized since it is a VEGF-ligand binding agent with 10 to 30% response as a monotherapy and 26 to 31% when used with interferon. The overall survival is 18 to 23 months with this therapy.[25] Other targeted agents such as temsirolimus and everolimus which are mammalian target of rapamycin (mTOR) inhibiting agents have been utilized, but IL-2 and sunitinib remain the mainstay of chemotherapy for advanced RCC.

Radiation Therapy

Historically, RCC has been considered radio resistant for the primary tumor, but metastatic RCC is routinely radiated for palliation.

Locoregional

Alternative to the cytoreductive nephrectomy, a complete embolization of the tumor within the kidney can be performed potentially saving some renal function. Use of bland embolization particles or ethanol is common. When ethanol is utilized, the procedure is extremely painful and monitored anesthesia care or general anesthetic is recommended. These patients commonly have the postembolization syndrome with nausea, vomiting, and flank pain causing them to be admitted to the hospital for 3 to 5 days. The use of intravenous steroids will diminish the edema in the embolized kidney and reduce the amount of pain medication needed. If the tumor is a large one, there is the potential of tumor lysis syndrome that is characterized by rapid development of hyperuricemia, hyperkalemia, hyperphosphatemia, hypocalcemia, and acute renal failure. The rapid death of tumor cells results in release of the intracellular contents into the circulation and injury to the renal tubules. Allopurinol is used to inhibit the nucleic acid byproducts to uric acid. It should be started orally at 600 mg/d a few days prior to the embolization.

RCC primary tumor has been embolized prior to surgery to help reduce hemorrhage. Additionally, embolization with radioactive ^{90}Y has been performed in a small number of patients. In this series of four patients, there were no recurrences in the 18-month follow-up. Difficulty in judging the exact dose to use was addressed by performing the ^{99m}Tc macroaggregated albumin (MAA) scan immediately before the radioembolization since the embolic effect of the MAA particles would change, however slightly, the accuracy of the shunt calculation. If too high a shunt is present, preliminary embolization with bland particles may be performed to cut down on the shunt before the isotope is administered.

RCC metastasizes to bone and is responsible for extraordinary bone pain. When the metastasis occurs in weight-bearing bones, the use of orthopaedic fixation devices can help prevent pathologic fractures. However, if the disease continues to grow and causes discomfort, several therapies are available. Since RCC and its bony metastases are hypervascular, both may be bland embolized to reduce any bleeding before surgery. Additionally, use of RFA to the lytic bone lesions is an excellent way to kill tumor but should be followed by augmentation with polymethylmethacrylate cement.

Prognosis at 5 years[26]:

- Stage I = 90%.
- Stage II = with T2a, 65 to 80%; with T2b, 50 to 70%.
- Stage III = with T3a, 40 to 65%; with T3b, 30 to 50%; with T3c, 20 to 40%.
- Stage IV = with T4, 0 to 20%; with M1, 0 to 10%.

References

1. Heck JE, Charbotel B, Moore LE, et al. Occupation and renal cell cancer in Central and Eastern Europe. Occup Environ Med 2010;67(1):47–53

2. Kovacs G, Akhtar M, Beckwith BJ, et al. The Heidelberg classification of renal cell tumours. J Pathol 1997;183(2):131–133

3. Linehan WM, Srinivasan R, Schmidt LS. The genetic basis of kidney cancer: a metabolic disease. Nat Rev Urol 2010;7(5):277–285

4. Nickerson ML, Warren MB, Toro JR, et al. Mutations in a novel gene lead to kidney tumors, lung wall defects, and benign tumors of the hair follicle in patients with the Birt-Hogg-Dubé syndrome. Cancer Cell 2002;2(2):157–164

5. Vanharanta S, Buchta M, McWhinney SR, et al. Early-onset renal cell carcinoma as a novel extraparaganglial component of SDHB-associated heritable paraganglioma. Am J Hum Genet 2004;74(1):153–159

6. Deng F-M, Melamed J, Zhou M. Pathology of renal cell carcinoma. In: Libertino JA, ed. Renal Cancer: Contemporary Management. New York, NY: Springer Science + Business Media; 2013:51–69

7. Gnarra JR, Tory K, Weng Y, et al. Mutations of the VHL tumour suppressor gene in renal carcinoma. Nat Genet 1994;7(1):85–90

8. Nickerson ML, Jaeger E, Shi Y, et al. Improved identification of von Hippel-Lindau gene alterations in clear cell renal tumors. Clin Cancer Res 2008;14(15):4726–4734

9. Farley MN, Schmidt LS, Mester JL, et al. A novel germline mutation in BAP1 predisposes to familial clear-cell renal cell carcinoma. Mol Cancer Res 2013;11(9):1061–1071

10. Dharmawardana PG, Giubellino A, Bottaro DP. Hereditary papillary renal carcinoma type I. Curr Mol Med 2004;4(8):855–868

11. Gad S, Lefèvre SH, Khoo SK, et al. Mutations in BHD and TP53 genes, but not in HNF1beta gene, in a large series of sporadic chromophobe renal cell carcinoma. Br J Cancer 2007;96(2):336–340

12. Nordstrom-O'Brien M, van der Luijt RB, van Rooijen E, et al. Genetic analysis of von Hippel-Lindau disease. Hum Mutat 2010;31(5):521–537

13. van Slegtenhorst M, de Hoogt R, Hermans C, et al. Identification of the tuberous sclerosis gene TSC1 on chromosome 9q34. Science 1997;277(5327):805–808

14. Bissler JJ, McCormack FX, Young LR, et al. Sirolimus for angiomyolipoma in tuberous sclerosis complex or lymphangioleiomyomatosis. N Engl J Med 2008;358(2):140–151

15. Chen HM, Fang JY. Genetics of the hamartomatous polyposis syndromes: a molecular review. Int J Colorectal Dis 2009;24(8):865–874

16. Rohan SM, Xiao Y, Liang Y, et al. Clear-cell papillary renal cell carcinoma: molecular and immunohistochemical analysis with emphasis on the von Hippel-Lindau gene and hypoxia-inducible factor pathway-related proteins. Mod Pathol 2011;24(9):1207–1220

17. Edge SB, Byrd DR, Compton CC. AJCC Cancer Staging Manual. 7th ed. New York, NY: Springer; 2010

18. Silverman SG, Israel GM, Herts BR, Richie JP. Management of the incidental renal mass. Radiology 2008;249(1):16–31

19. Atwell TD, Schmit GD, Boorjian SA, et al. Percutaneous ablation of renal masses measuring 3.0 cm and smaller: comparative local control and complications after radiofrequency ablation and cryoablation. AJR Am J Roentgenol 2013;200(2):461–466

20. Van Poppel H, Becker F, Cadeddu JA, et al. Treatment of localised renal cell carcinoma. Eur Urol 2011;60(4):662–672

21. Volpe A, Cadeddu JA, Cestari A, et al. Contemporary management of small renal masses. Eur Urol 2011;60(3):501–515

22. Lopez Hänninen E, Kirchner H, Atzpodien J. Interleukin-2 based home therapy of metastatic renal cell carcinoma: risks and benefits in 215 consecutive single institution patients. J Urol 1996;155(1):19–25

23. McDermott DF, Drake CG, Sznol M, et al. Clinical activity and safety of anti-PD-1 (BMS-936558, MDX-1106) in patients with previously treated metastatic renal cell carcinoma (mRCC). J Clin Oncol 2012;30(15, Suppl):4505

24. Motzer RJ, Hutson TE, Tomczak P, et al. Sunitinib versus interferon alfa in metastatic renal-cell carcinoma. N Engl J Med 2007;356(2):115–124

25. Bukowski RM, Kabbinavar FF, Figlin RA, et al. Randomized phase II study of erlotinib combined with bevacizumab compared with bevacizumab alone in metastatic renal cell cancer. J Clin Oncol 2007;25(29):4536–4541

26. Lane BR, Kattan MW. Prognostic models and algorithms in renal cell carcinoma. Urol Clin North Am 2008;35(4):613–625, vii

14   Urothelial Cancer and Transitional Cell Cancer

Douglas M. Coldwell

Epidemiology

Urothelial cancers are more common in men than in women. The incidence of these tumors is increasing. Risk factors include gene abnormalities, chemical exposure, and chronic irritation. No single gene can predict the presence of this tumor, but there are a plethora of genetic abnormalities that occur with this tumor. Chemical exposure to aromatic amines, aniline dyes, tobacco use, and nitrites/nitrates have been associated with the development of bladder cancers. Chronic irritation from indwelling catheters, recurrent urinary tract infections, Schistosoma haematobium, and irradiation have also been noted to be initiating agents.[1–4]

Pathology

About 95% are transitional cell cancer (TCC) with the other 5% either squamous or adenocarcinoma. Most TCCs occur in the bladder and the remaining 10% in the renal pelvis with fewer than 2% in the ureter.

For bladder cancer, the functional pathology is centered on whether the tumor is confined to the epithelium (stage Ta) or has invaded the lamina proprium (stage T1). These tumors can be managed endoscopically but have a recurrence rate of at least 50% at 5 years.[5]

Cytologic Characteristics

- G1 = Low grade.
- G2 = Intermediate grade.
- G3 = High grade.

Genetics

Epidermal growth factor receptor (*EGFR*), including *EGFR1* and *EGFR2*, and vascular endothelial growth factor (*VEGR*) are produced by most bladder tumors. The degree of overexpression of these products are indicative of an unfavorable outcome. Since there are targeted drugs to these mutations, inhibition of them may have a tumoricidal effect. The altered expression of *p53*, *p16*, and *pRB* are of no prognostic significance, but the overexpression of human epidermal growth factor receptor 2 (HER2) suggested an inferior response rate to therapy, while EGFR overexpress was associated with an improved response. Additionally, higher levels of *VEGF* and *cyclooxygenase-2* are associated with disease progression.[6,7]

Staging[8]

Tumor

- Ta = Noninvasive papillary carcinoma.
- T1 = Tumor invades lamina propria only.
- T2 = Tumor invades muscularis propria.
- pT2a = Tumor invades inner half of superficial muscle.
- pT2b = Tumor invades out half of deep muscle.
- T3 = Tumor invades perivesical tissue.
- pT3a = Invasion is microscopic.
- pT3b = Invasion is macroscopic with extravesical mass.
- T4 = Invades prostatic stroma, uterus, vagina, pelvis or abdominal wall.
- T4a = Invades prostate, uterus, vagina.
- T4b = Invades pelvic or abdominal wall.

Lymph Nodes

- N1 = Tumor in a single lymph node in primary drainage region.
- N2 = Metastasis in multiple lymph nodes in primary drainage region.
- N3 = Common iliac lymph node involvement.

Metastases

- M0 = No distant metastases.
- M1 = Distant metastases.

In patients with bladder cancer, 70% have Ta or T1 disease with 15 to 20% of these progressing to T2 disease. In patients with Ta or T1 disease, 50 to 70% will recur after therapy. If the tumor is G1 or G2 and Ta, there is a lower recurrence rate at 50% and a 5% progression rate. However, in high-risk disease, G3, with T1 or multifocal disease there is a higher recurrence rate at 70% and a 30 to 50% progression rate to T2 or higher.[9] Patients at risk for developing a transition to a higher grade tumor, that is, those with G3 tumors, following treatment with a transurethral resection of bladder tumor (TURBT) are usually treated with intravesical drug therapy. These highly irritating agents, for example, bacillus Calmette–Guérin (BCG), interferon, mitomycin C, and gemcitabine, may cause bladder contracture, dysuria. There has been no conclusive study to validate the use of this technique.[10–12]

In patients with T1 BCG-refractory disease, a cystectomy is indicated. Patients with G3 T1 disease are often initially treated with a cystectomy due to the high rate of progression through the muscularis propria citing results of a 10-year cancer-specific survival of 80% when this technique is used when the G3 T1 disease is discovered and only 50% when the cystectomy is performed after the tumor has penetrated the muscularis mucosa.[13,14]

Treatment

Surgery

Surgical approaches include abdominal or orthotopic continent diversions. The abdominal diversion needs a valve and the patient catheterizes himself every 4 hours. The orthotopic diversion utilizes the bladder sphincter to maintain continence with voiding by using the Valsalva maneuver. Incontinent diversions utilize a segment of small bowel with one end brought to the skin as an ostomy and the ureters implanted on the other. Complications may include urine leak, fistulas, anastomotic stenosis, metabolic acidosis, decreased renal function, renal calculi, and sepsis. The mechanical strictures may be addressed by placement of nephrostomy catheters, indwelling ureteral stents, and stents that are curled in the renal pelvis and extend to the ostomy bag. All these stents are placed by interventional radiology (IR) and usually require routine exchange to prevent obstruction.[15–17]

Chemotherapy

The standard cisplatin containing regimes for TCC are methotrexate, vinblastine, doxorubicin, and cisplatin (MVAC) with a response rate of 40 to 65% and a median survival of 12 to 14 months.[18,19] Cisplatin, methotrexate, and vinblastine (CMV) has a response rate of 36% and a median survival of 7 months, while gemcitabine and cisplatin have a response rate of 49% and a median survival of 14 months.[20] In patients who are ineligible to receive cisplatin due to medical comorbidities, the combination of gemcitabine and carboplatin demonstrates an equivalent survival to that seen in MVAC but is better tolerated and has a better safety profile. Gemcitabine and paclitaxel may also be considered in patients who cannot receive platinum-based chemotherapy with a survival of 14 months, which is comparable to gemcitabine/carboplatin.[21]

Radiation Therapy

Recent advances in the use of radiation therapy to control T2 disease have increased the bladder preservation rate. The long-term survival of 64% with T2 tumors and 22% with T3/T4 tumors is attractive. Additional studies combining TURBT with chemoradiotherapy have improved local control even more. If the patient has a clinical complete response to radiotherapy, they should be considered for bladder conservation therapy. However, up to 30% will develop more invasive tumors and require a radical cystectomy.[22]

Locoregional Therapy

The use of nephrostomy tubes, indwelling stents, and stents within incontinent pouches is commonly performed in IR. The nephrostomy tubes and stents in the pouches must be regularly changed to prevent occlusion and sepsis. A regular schedule of changes every 2 to 3 months is recommended. Close cooperation with the urology service is necessary to coordinate the care on these patients.

Prognosis

After a radical cystectomy, in pathologic stage pTa, T1 G3, 10-year survival is 82% cancer-specific survival. While if the stage is pT2, pN0, the survival is 73% and if the stage is pT3–pT4a or pN1–pN2 it is 33%. If any lymph nodes are positive, the 10-year survival decreases to 28%.[23-27] The biology of the upper tract TCC tumors is considered to be identical to that seen in the bladder.

Role of Interventional Radiology

IR techniques are used not only for management of the nephrostomy tubes, ureteral stents, and the urine drainage, but also to biopsy local recurrence, embolize, or utilize intra-arterial infusion of chemotherapy in several different types of genitourinary tumors. This may be used particularly in the management of recurrent squamous cell carcinoma after chemoradiation therapy.[28,29]

References

1. Siegel R, Naishadham D, Jemal A. Cancer statistics, 2013. CA Cancer J Clin 2013;63(1):11–30

2. Munoz JJ, Ellison LM. Upper tract urothelial neoplasms: incidence and survival during the last 2 decades. J Urol 2000;164(5):1523–1525

3. Jelaković B, Karanović S, Vuković-Lela I, et al. Aristolactam-DNA adducts are a biomarker of environmental exposure to aristolochic acid. Kidney Int 2012;81(6):559–567

4. Solomon DA, Kim JS, Bondaruk J, et al. Frequent truncating mutations of STAG2 in bladder cancer. Nat Genet 2013;45(12):1428–1430

5. Younes M, Sussman J, True LD. The usefulness of the level of the muscularis mucosae in the staging of invasive transitional cell carcinoma of the urinary bladder. Cancer 1990;66(3):543–548

6. Ciardiello F, Caputo R, Bianco R, et al. Antitumor effect and potentiation of cytotoxic drugs activity in human cancer cells by ZD-1839 (Iressa), an epidermal growth factor receptor-selective tyrosine kinase inhibitor. Clin Cancer Res 2000;6(5):2053–2063

7. Jimenez RE, Hussain M, Bianco FJ Jr, et al. Her-2/neu overexpression in muscle-invasive urothelial carcinoma of the bladder: prognostic significance and comparative analysis in primary and metastatic tumors. Clin Cancer Res 2001;7(8):2440–2447

8. Edge SB, Byrd DR, Compton CC. AJCC Cancer Staging Manual. 7th ed. New York, NY: Springer; 2010

9. Gray PJ, Lin CC, Jemal A, et al. Clinical-pathologic stage discrepancy in bladder cancer patients treated with radical cystectomy: results from the national cancer data base. Int J Radiat Oncol Biol Phys 2014;88(5):1048–1056

10. Di Stasi SM, Valenti M, Verri C, et al. Electromotive instillation of mitomycin immediately before transurethral resection for patients with primary urothelial non-muscle invasive bladder cancer: a randomised controlled trial. Lancet Oncol 2011;12(9):871–879

11. Lamm DL, Blumenstein BA, Crissman JD, et al. Maintenance bacillus Calmette-Guerin immunotherapy for recurrent TA, T1 and carcinoma in situ transitional cell carcinoma of the bladder: a randomized Southwest Oncology Group Study. J Urol 2000;163(4):1124–1129

12. Oddens J, Brausi M, Sylvester R, et al. Final results of an EORTC-GU cancers group randomized study of maintenance bacillus Calmette-Guérin in intermediate- and high-risk Ta, T1 papillary carcinoma of the urinary bladder: one-third dose versus full dose and 1 year versus 3 years of maintenance. Eur Urol 2013;63(3):462–472

13. Yiou R, Patard JJ, Benhard H, Abbou CC, Chopin DK. Outcome of radical cystectomy for bladder cancer according to the disease type at presentation. BJU Int 2002;89(4):374–378

14. Gray PJ, Shipley WU, Efstathiou JA, Zietman AL. Recent advances and the emerging role for chemoradiation in nonmuscle invasive bladder cancer. Curr Opin Urol 2013;23(5):429–434

15. McDougal WS. Metabolic complications of urinary intestinal diversion. J Urol 1992;147(5):1199–1208

16. Eisenberg MS, Thompson RH, Frank I, et al. Long-term renal function outcomes after radical cystectomy. J Urol 2014;191(3):619–625

17. Chahal R, Sundaram SK, Iddenden R, Forman DF, Weston PM, Harrison SC. A study of the morbidity, mortality and long-term survival following radical cystectomy and radical radiotherapy in the treatment of invasive bladder cancer in Yorkshire. Eur Urol 2003;43(3):246–257

18. Herr HW. Outcome of patients who refuse cystectomy after receiving neoadjuvant chemotherapy for muscle-invasive bladder cancer. Eur Urol 2008;54(1):126–132

19. Black PC, Brown GA, Grossman HB, Dinney CP. Neoadjuvant chemotherapy for bladder cancer. World J Urol 2006;24(5):531–542

20. Hall RR. Neoadjuvant cisplatin, methotrexate, and vinblastine chemotherapy for muscle-invasive bladder cancer: a randomized controlled trial. International collaboration of trialists. Lancet 1999;354(9178):533–540

21. Bellmunt J, von der Maase H, Mead GM, et al. Randomized phase III study comparing paclitaxel/cisplatin/gemcitabine and gemcitabine/cisplatin in patients with locally advanced or metastatic urothelial cancer without prior systemic therapy: EORTC Intergroup Study 30987. J Clin Oncol 2012;30(10):1107–1113

22. Gakis G, Efstathiou J, Lerner SP, et al; International Consultation on Urologic Disease-European Association of Urology Consultation on Bladder Cancer 2012. ICUD-EAU International Consultation on Bladder Cancer 2012: Radical cystectomy and bladder preservation for muscle-invasive urothelial carcinoma of the bladder. Eur Urol 2013;63(1):45–57

23. Gschwend JE, Dahm P, Fair WR. Disease specific survival as endpoint of outcome for bladder cancer patients following radical cystectomy. Eur Urol 2002;41(4):440–448

24. Stein JP, Cai J, Groshen S, Skinner DG. Risk factors for patients with pelvic lymph node metastases following radical cystectomy with en bloc pelvic lymphadenectomy: concept of lymph node density. J Urol 2003;170(1):35–41

25. Stein JP, Lieskovsky G, Cote R, et al. Radical cystectomy in the treatment of invasive bladder cancer: long-term results in 1,054 patients. J Clin Oncol 2001;19(3):666–675

26. Dalbagni G, Genega E, Hashibe M, et al. Cystectomy for bladder cancer: a contemporary series. J Urol 2001;165(4):1111–1116

27. Grossman HB, Natale RB, Tangen CM, et al. Neoadjuvant chemotherapy plus cystectomy compared with cystectomy alone for locally advanced bladder cancer. N Engl J Med 2003;349(9):859–866

28. Roth AD, Berney CR, Rohner S, et al. Intra-arterial chemotherapy in locally advanced or recurrent carcinomas of the penis and anal canal: an active treatment modality with curative potential. Br J Cancer 2000;83(12):1637–1642

29. Liu JY, Li YH, Liu ZW, et al. Intraarterial chemotherapy with gemcitabine and cisplatin in locally advanced or recurrent penile squamous cell carcinoma. Chin J Cancer 2013;32(11):619–623

15   Prostate Cancer

Douglas M. Coldwell

Epidemiology

Almost all cases of prostate cancer (PC) occur in men over the age of 50 years. Having a first-degree relative (father or brother) increases the risk two- to threefold, having two first-degree relatives increases it 5-fold to 11-fold.[1] In the United States, PC is more common in African American men than in white men. It is also associated with diet, hypertension, obesity, lack of activity, a high number of sexual partners, and sexually transmitted diseases.[2]

Pathology

Adenocarcinoma arising from the acinar and proximal duct epithelium in the peripheral zone of the prostate making early extracapsular extension frequent. It is multifocal in 85% of cases.[3,4] Pathologic grading on Gleason's scale is an important factor in the prognosis and treatment recommendations. The score of the dominant (>50%) of the biopsy specimen is determined and then added to the score of the next greatest type, as in "Gleason 4+3":

- Gleason 1 = Very close to normal without invasion into normal tissue (rarely seen).
- Gleason 2 = Glands are looser and not as uniform as in 1 (rarely seen).
- Gleason 3 = Clearly infiltrative neoplasm with invasion into adjacent normal tissue. Glands are irregular in size but can be circumscribed.
- Gleason 4 = Glands are fused together with no clear separation with scalloped edges
- Gleason 5 = No glandular differentiation and composed of sheets of cells or solid cords or individual cells. No round glands are present.[5–7]

Most treatable lesions are of Gleason scores of 5 to 7 with the biopsy obtained after an abnormal serum prostate-specific antigen or digital rectal examination. Tumors of Gleason scores of 8 to 10 are advanced lesions where likely only palliative care is given.

Genetics

Diagnosis

Screening is a controversial subject. Serum prostate-specific antigen (PSA) levels are not recommended by the United States Preventative Services Task Force due to the overdiagnosis and overtreatment of PC without increasing overall survival (OS) and most of the cancers diagnosed would be asymptomatic.[8] Unfortunately, the screening cannot discriminate between the aggressive tumors and those that are low grade and unlikely to become aggressive. Given that imaging and serial digital prostate exams are the best ways to detect PC, any suspicious nodule on digital exam should be followed up by a magnetic resonance imaging (MRI) and any suspicious lesions biopsied. Elderly patients or patients with an expected life span of less than 10 years should not be screened. These lesions are graded by the Prostate Imaging - Reporting and Data System (PI-RADS). The latest version, PI-RADSv2, is focused on detection of significant PC, which is Gleason grade 4 or higher with a volume greater than 0.5 mL. The MRI parameters are spelled out in detail in the American College of Radiology publication.[9,10] The PI-RADS score ranges from 1 to 5:

- 1 = Most likely benign.
- 2 = Clinically significant PC is unlikely to be present.
- 3 = Presence of PC is equivocal.
- 4 = PC is likely to be present.
- 5 = PC is highly likely to be present.

Staging[11]

Tumor

- T1 = Clinically inapparent. Neither palpable nor present on imaging.
- T2 = Palpable or visible tumor within the prostate.
- T2a = Less than half of one lobe.
- T2b = More than half of one lobe, not both.
- T2c = Both lobes.
- T3 = Tumor extends through prostate capsule.
- T3a = Extracapsular extension.
- T3b = Seminal vesical involvement.
- T4 = Tumor is fixed or invades adjacent structures other than seminal vesicles.

Lymph Nodes

In intermediate-risk PC with a Gleason score of 7 to 8, 5 to 10% of patients have pelvic lymph node involvement, while those with high-risk PC with a Gleason score of greater than 8 have a 20 to 50% risk.

Metastases

Metastases occur predominantly in bones and lymph nodes but occasionally to liver where it is a hypervascular tumor.

Treatment

Treatment is dependent on the clinical stage, PSA level, Gleason score, age of patient, and presence of metastatic disease.

Clinically Localized Disease

Active surveillance is recommended in those patients who have localized disease that is low grade, PSA < 10, and Gleason score 6, and in younger patients. The repeat MRI should be obtained every 2 years with the PSA level. The psychological effect of knowing that a low-grade tumor is present but nothing is "being treated" is difficult for many patients. Approximately 20% of the active surveillance patients elect to undergo surgery or radiation therapy after 1 year. In patients with low-risk PC, when the doubling time of the PSA is less than 2 years, OS with active surveillance at 8 years is reported to be 85% and disease-specific and metastasis-free survival to be 99%. About 25% of patients were treated by 5 years and 40% by 10 years with the delay associated with a lack of cancer control suggesting that waiting until the PSA doubling time reached 2 years was too late.[12] Patients undergoing active surveillance followed by serial biopsies and intervention determined by the change in biopsy score were treated at a mean of 6.5 years with 40% by 5 years and 59% by 10 years. These patients demonstrated that the delay in therapy did not affect cancer control.[13] These results suggest that diagnosis by PSA alone is insufficient and under-grade the tumor, and serial biopsies are far better at determining the time of intervention. Most physicians are utilizing MRI to follow active surveillance patients with early biopsies.

Surgery

Radical prostatectomy (RP) is an option to active surveillance. The success of the procedure to obtain an R0 resection is due to the experience and skill of the performing urologist. RP compared with watchful waiting (as opposed to active surveillance) reduced the risk of death from PC by 44%, the clinical local recurrence by 66%, and the need for anti-androgenic therapy by 51%.[14] In a large U.S. trial, men with clinically localized PC were randomized to either observation or RP. The study showed that the risk of dying from PC when an RP was performed in aggressive cancers with a PSA > 10 or had aggressive histologic features was reduced and the likelihood of metastases was decreased.[15] This suggests that those patients who undergo RP with an intermediate- or high-risk PC have less risk of metastases and of death when early RP is utilized. Even in those patients who have a Gleason score of 8 to 10, RP has a 42% probability of progression-free survival at 10 years.[16]

The most important complications after surgery are incontinence and impotence. Nerve-sparing surgery should decrease the rate of impotence, but the size of the tumor and the experience of the surgeon are the critical determinants. Rates of impotence of 30 to 80% have been reported and incontinence of 16%.[17]

Radiation Therapy

Use of external beam radiation therapy, intensity-modulated radiation therapy (IMRT), or brachytherapy with implanted radioactive seeds is also used as a monotherapy for PC. The target dose to the tumor should be at least 75 Gy and preferably 80 Gy in higher risk patients.[18] The 1-year risk of impotence after external beam radiotherapy has been reported to be 42%[19] Brachytherapy seed implantation has been demonstrated to have an equivalent rate of tumor control to external beam radiation and to surgery without the rates of initial complications. These seeds are either ^{103}Pd or ^{125}I; both are low-energy gamma emitters so that the tumor receives a dose of at least 80 Gy. The 10-year tumor control rate is 95% and a rate of impotence of 1% at 1 year and incontinence of 10% at 1 year. However, the rates of both increase so that at 7 years the rate of impotence is 70 to 80% and incontinence is 20%.[20] Brachytherapy is utilized in patients who have significant percentage of disease in biopsies, increasing PSA velocity, or a dominant lesion demonstrated on MRI. Brachytherapy is preferred over IMRT since it is a single treatment. In larger treatment volumes, androgen deprivation therapy (ADT) is used for 3 to 4 months to decrease the size of the prostate by 30 to 40%.

In high-risk patients who have received an RP, adjuvant radiation therapy has shown to be advantageous with a PFS rate of 40 versus 60% in observation-only patients and the 10-year PC mortality was 3.9 versus 5.4%, respectively.[21]

Chemotherapy

Androgen deprivation therapy (ADT) has been utilized since the 1940s as a chemical castration to retard the growth of PC. Currently, its use is primarily in locally advanced PC as an adjunct to radiation, in a neo-adjuvant or adjuvant, or concurrent role. When ADT is combined with at least 70-Gy external beam radiation therapy (EBRT), the results are significantly better.[22–24]

In advanced PC, docetaxel has been shown to prolong OS when compared with any docetaxel-based doublet chemotherapy.[25] In single-agent therapies, docetaxel demonstrates a 19-month OS when used as first-line therapy, which has not been statistically exceeded by any other doublet therapies. Other agents, such as [223]Ra have been targeted to palliate the pain of bone metastases. EBRT has also been utilized to target bony metastases, but it takes 6 weeks to become effective and has about a 60 to 70% response rate.

With this plethora of treatments, the choices are dependent on the size of the lesion, presence of extraprostatic disease, patient preferences, and clinical evaluation. When metastases are present, ADT can assist in their management. When this therapy is instituted, most PSA levels will return to normal, the measurable tumor masses will decrease in size by at least half, the bone metastases will decrease in size as measured on bone scan, and patient's symptoms will improve in a majority. Complete response of the tumor with ADT is unlikely. The number of bone metastases is also directly proportional to the survival rate.

In patients who are androgen deprivation or castration resistant, the treatment becomes more complex. In the pre-PSA era, prednisone was shown to be effective in treating the pain of bone metastases. Mitoxantrone was developed from this experience and was the only therapy used as a doublet with prednisone. Consequently, docetaxel and its successor, cabazitaxel, have been shown to be effective in the treatment of these patients showing OS of 13 to 15 months. Both the prednisone and the ADT agents result in osteoporosis, increasing the risks of fracture and further bone pain. Denosumab is a monoclonal antibody inhibiting osteoclast function that reduces bone loss and fracture rate as well as an increase in time to the development of bone metastases.[26,27]

Locoregional Therapy

High-intensity focused ultrasound is currently being evaluated for clinical efficacy. The high-energy ultrasound waves are focused on to the tumor and it is heated above 50°C. The treatment is administered under ultrasound guidance via a transrectal probe. This treatment is touted as an outpatient treatment but lasts about 3 hours depending on the size of the prostate being ablated. A recent study demonstrated its use in 41 men who received this treatment and a targeted biopsy on the tumor site 1 year later. In all, 77% of these patients had no evidence of tumor and there were fewer genitourinary side effects than surgery.[28]

Cryotherapy has been utilized with several probes inserted through the perineum into the prostate. The impotency rate is 90% immediately since no protection for the nervous structures is possible. It is utilized in patients to whom sexual function is not important, in salvage therapy in patients who have failed brachytherapy, or in young patients with discrete focal disease.[29]

Prostate Embolization for Prostatic Hyperplasia

The other major tumor in the prostate is benign prostatic hyperplasia (BPH), an enlargement of the prostate through the growth of nodules of stromal and epithelial cells in the transitional zone, seen in men over 50 years of age and causes urinary retention, difficulty and frequency of urination. BPH may also cause a rise in the PSA level but is not a precancerous condition. Androgens play a critical role but are not the cause of BPH. Dihydrotestosterone is a metabolite of testosterone by the enzyme 5α reductase that primarily exists in the stromal cells and acts on the circulating testosterone. Dihydrotestosterone is a growth mediator and is then concentrated in the stromal cells causing them to multiply, while selective α-1 blockers and the 5α-reductase inhibitor, finasteride, are utilized for treatment. These medical treatments may not be effective or have unacceptable side effects in many patients.

A new application for arterial embolization is being investigated, the bland embolization of the prostate. The arterial anatomy is reasonably consistent with a single prostatic artery per side in 57% of patients with the remaining 43% having two arteries. Most of these arteries are branches of the internal pudendal artery (56%) with other origins making up the remainder, common anterior gluteal–pudendal trunk (28%), obturator artery (12%), and the inferior gluteal artery (4%).[30–32] Embolization is performed to stasis with either coils or 100- to 200-µ-diameter polyvinyl alcohol foam particles. The patients were taken off their medical therapy for the BPH before the embolization. Technical success occurred in 98% of patients and few reported any pain either during or following the procedure. Patients reported an improvement in their lower urinary tract symptoms within hours of the procedure and most within a few weeks. The clinical success rate was 85% at short-term follow-up, 81% at medium-term, and 76% at long-term (6-year) follow-up.[33]

The results of embolization for BPH are excellent, which suggest that embolization with chemotherapy added to the embolization mixture may have a role in the direct therapy of unresectable PC or downgrading the tumor mass by cytoreduction. Investigation into this potential new therapy for PC is in the initial investigation phase.

Radio Frequency Ablation for Bone Metastases

PC commonly metastasizes to bone usually in the form of sclerotic lesions. These painful tumors are often treated by administration of systemic radiation that localizes in bone, for example, ^{223}Ra, but it is very expensive and not always available. With the advent of purpose-designed Radiofrequency Ablation (RFA) catheters for bone, it is straightforward to place the bone guiding catheter in the affected bone followed by the placement of the RFA probe. Since these tumors are extremely dense, the placement of the bone guiding needle can be very difficult and a hand or power drill is an essential aid. After the placement of the RFA probe, the generator is started at its lowest power level for several minutes before any increase in power is made. The increase in power is made very slowly so that there is a bigger "burn" before the probe "impedes out." This refers to the fact that the generators are constant power generators and, as the tumor temperature increases, the resistance to the flow of alternating current field increases linearly. This forces the current applied to decrease by the square to keep the power constant from the equation: $P = I^2R$, a form of Ohm's law. The tumor heats slowly and may impede out several times before adequate therapy is applied. But by just repeatedly letting the tumor cool slightly and re-energizing the RFA probe, the tumor will eventually become hot enough to cause tissue damage. Because the tumor is so dense, no polymethyl methacrylate (PMMA) cement is able to be intercalated into the tumor. The RFA probe may be used by itself to obtain pain relief in these patients with sclerotic metastases.

Lytic metastases are treated similarly. But these will more easily heat to thermal destructive temperature and the PMMA cement instilled so that it can intercalate into the bone. Extravasation of cement may occur:

- Laterally extending to the neural foramen causing local pain, anteriorly and enter Batson's plexus resulting in a pulmonary embolus.
- Superiorly or inferiorly with little to no effect.
- Posteriorly solidifying in the spinal canal potentially resulting in spinal cord irritation.

However, it is unusual to have the extravasation posteriorly if the posterior wall of the vertebral body is intact and especially since the placement of the cement is performed under lateral fluoroscopy, and the instillation of the cement can be quickly stopped if the boundary of the cement approaches the posterior margin of the vertebral body. Additionally, a midline osteotome may be utilized to direct the cement along the destroyed posterior wall to form a dam so that the cement infused more anteriorly will not be able to pass into the spinal canal. This is only possible with the very thick cement and the very stiff and curving osteotome.

References

1. Smith JR, Freije D, Carpten JD, et al. Major susceptibility locus for prostate cancer on chromosome 1 suggested by a genome-wide search. Science 1996;274(5291):1371–1374

2. Vertosick EA, Poon BY, Vickers AJ. Relative value of race, family history and prostate specific antigen as indications for early initiation of prostate cancer screening. J Urol 2014;192(3):724–728

3. DeMarzo AM, Nelson WG, Isaacs WB, Epstein JI. Pathological and molecular aspects of prostate cancer. Lancet 2003;361(9361):955–964

4. Nelson WG, De Marzo AM, Isaacs WB. Prostate cancer. N Engl J Med 2003;349(4):366–381

5. Fleming ID, Cooper JS, Henson DE, et al. American Joint Committee on Cancer. AJCC Cancer Staging Manual. 5th ed. Philadelphia, PA: JB Lippincott; 1997

6. Gleason DF. Classification of prostatic carcinomas. Cancer Chemother Rep 1966;50(3):125–128

7. Gleason DF, Mellinger GT. Prediction of prognosis for prostatic adeno-carcinoma by combined histological grading and clinical staging. J Urol 1974;111(1):58–64

8. Moyer VA; U.S. Preventive Services Task Force. Screening for prostate cancer: U.S. Preventive Services Task Force recommendation statement. Ann Intern Med 2012;157(2):120–134

9. Barentsz JO, Weinreb JC, Verma S, et al. Synopsis of the PI-RADS v2 Guidelines for Multiparametric Prostate Magnetic Resonance Imaging and Recommendations for Use. Eur Urol 2016;69(1):41–49

10. http://www.acr.org/Quality-Safety/Resources/PIRADS-PI-RADS, Prostate Imaging Reporting and Data System, version 2. Last accessed June 13, 2017.

11. Edge S, Byrd DR, Compton CC, et al. American Joint Committee on Cancer. AJCC Cancer Staging Manual. 7th ed. New York, NY: Springer; 2010

12. Klotz L, Zhang L, Lam A, Nam R, Mamedov A, Loblaw A. Clinical results of long-term follow-up of a large, active surveillance cohort with localized prostate cancer. J Clin Oncol 2010;28(1):126–131

13. Mullins JK, Bonekamp D, Landis P, et al. Multiparametric magnetic resonance imaging findings in men with low-risk prostate cancer followed using active surveillance. BJU Int 2013;111(7):1037–1045

14. Bill-Axelson A, Holmberg L, Garmo H, et al. Radical prostatectomy or watchful waiting in early prostate cancer. N Engl J Med 2014;370(10):932–942

15. Wilt TJ, Brawer MK, Jones KM, et al; Prostate Cancer Intervention versus Observation Trial (PIVOT) Study Group. Radical prostatectomy versus observation for localized prostate cancer. N Engl J Med 2012;367(3):203–213

16. Yossepowitch O, Eggener SE, Serio AM, et al. Secondary therapy, metastatic progression, and cancer-specific mortality in men with clinically high-risk prostate cancer treated with radical prostatectomy. Eur Urol 2008;53(5):950–959

17. Kaplan JR, Lee Z, Eun DD, Reese AC. Complications of minimally invasive surgery and their management. Curr Urol Rep 2016;17(6):47

18. Beckendorf V, Guerif S, Le Prisé E, et al. 70 Gy versus 80 Gy in localized prostate cancer: 5-year results of GETUG 06 randomized trial. Int J Radiat Oncol Biol Phys 2011;80(4):1056–1063

19. Cozzarini C, Rancati T, Badenchini F, et al. Baseline status and dose to the penile bulb predict impotence 1 year after radiotherapy for prostate cancer. Strahlenther Onkol 2016;192(5):297–304

20. Putora PM, Engeler D, Haile SR, et al. Erectile function following brachytherapy, external beam radiotherapy, or radical prostatectomy in prostate cancer patients. Strahlenther Onkol 2016;192(3):182–189

21. Bolla M, van Poppel H, Tombal B, et al; European Organisation for Research and Treatment of Cancer, Radiation Oncology and Genito-Urinary Groups. Postoperative radiotherapy after radical prostatectomy for high-risk prostate cancer: long-term results of a randomised controlled trial (EORTC trial 22911). Lancet 2012;380(9858):2018–2027

22. D'Amico AV. Radiation and hormonal therapy for locally advanced and clinically localized prostate cancer. Urology 2002; 60(3, Suppl 1):32–37, discussion 37–38

23. Jones CU, Hunt D, McGowan DG, et al. Radiotherapy and short-term androgen deprivation for localized prostate cancer. N Engl J Med 2011;365(2):107–118

24. Lee AK. Radiation therapy combined with hormone therapy for prostate cancer. Semin Radiat Oncol 2006;16(1):20–28

25. Tannock IF, de Wit R, Berry WR, et al; TAX 327 Investigators. Docetaxel plus prednisone or mitoxantrone plus prednisone for advanced prostate cancer. N Engl J Med 2004;351(15):1502–1512

26. Fizazi K, Carducci M, Smith M, et al. Denosumab versus zoledronic acid for treatment of bone metastases in men with castration-resistant prostate cancer: a randomised, double-blind study. Lancet 2011;377(9768):813–822

27. Smith MR, Saad F, Egerdie B, et al. Effects of denosumab on bone mineral density in men receiving androgen deprivation therapy for prostate cancer. J Urol 2009;182(6):2670–2675

28. Jácome-Pita F, Sánchez-Salas R, Barret E, Amaruch N, Gonzalez-Enguita C, Cathelineau X. Focal therapy in prostate cancer: the current situation. Ecancermedicalscience 2014;8:435

29. Rukstalis D, Katz A. A Handbook of Urologic Cryoablation. Boca Raton, FL: CRC Press; 2007

30. Bilhim T, Casal D, Furtado A, Pais D, O'Neill JE, Pisco JM. Branching patterns of the male internal iliac artery: imaging findings. Surg Radiol Anat 2011;33(2):151–159

31. Bilhim T, Pisco JM, Furtado A, et al. Prostatic arterial supply: demonstration by multirow detector angio CT and catheter angiography. Eur Radiol 2011;21(5):1119–1126

32. Bilhim T, Pisco JM, Rio Tinto H, et al. Prostatic arterial supply: anatomic and imaging findings relevant for selective arterial embolization. J Vasc Interv Radiol 2012;23(11):1403–1415

33. Pisco JM, Bilhim T, Pinheiro LC, et al. Medium- and long-term outcome of prostate artery embolization for patients with benign prostatic hyperplasia: results in 630 patients. J Vasc Interv Radiol 2016;27(8):1115–1122

16 Breast Cancer

Douglas M. Coldwell

Epidemiology

Breast cancer is the most frequent cancer in women and the second most frequent cause of cancer death in women. It is more frequent in industrialized nations than in developing ones, but the rates in the former are decreasing likely due to screening and the rates in the latter are rising.

Pathology

Breast cancer usually arises in the terminal duct lobule. It is classified by light microscopy as either lobular or ductal. The most common type is invasive or infiltrating ductal carcinoma (70–80%). The remaining 20 to 30% are subtypes that must represent at least 90% of the tumor.[1]

Genetics

Familial breast cancer comprises 20 to 30% of all breast cancers. *BRCA1* and *BRCA2* are the two genes associated with familial breast and ovarian cancer syndrome, which is about half of all inherited breast cancers. About 70 to 80% of breast cancer is sporadic and not associated with a particular genetic alteration.[2,3] If either *BRCA1* or *BRCA2* is present, there is a 60 to 85% lifetime risk of breast cancer and a 15 to 40% risk of ovarian cancer. The tumors associated with the *BRCA1* or *BRCA2* mutation are likely to be estrogen receptor (ER) and progesterone receptor negative (PR negative) and overexpress human epidermal growth factor receptor 2 (*HER2*).

Other hereditary syndromes include the following:

- Li–Fraumeni syndrome = Breast cancer, soft-tissue sarcoma, CNS (central nervous system) tumors, adrenocortical cancer, leukemia, and prostate cancer. Risk of breast cancer is 50 to 90% by the age of 50 years. Genetic mutation is *TP53* (tumor protein 53).
- Cowden's syndrome = Breast cancers, hamartoma, thyroid, oral mucosa, endometrial brain tumors. Risk of breast cancer is 25 to 50%. Genetic mutation is *PTEN* (phosphate and tensin homolog).

- Familial diffuse gastric cancer = Lobular breast cancer, gastric cancer. Incidence of breast cancer is at least six times normal. Genetic mutation is *CDH1* (cadherin-1).
- Peutz–Jeghers syndrome = Breast, ovarian, testis, pancreas, cervix, uterine, colon cancers; melanocytic macules of lips and digits; gastrointestinal hamartomatous polyps. Breast cancer risk is 30 to 50% by the age of 70 years. Genetic mutation is *STK11* (serine/threonine kinase 11)/*LKB1* (liver kinase B1).[4]

Staging[5]

Tumor

- Tis = Tumor in situ.
- T1 = Tumor is less than 2 cm in greatest dimension.
- T2 = Tumor is between 2 and 5 cm in greatest dimension.
- T3 = Tumor is greater than 5 cm in greatest dimension.
- T4a = Extension to chest wall.
- T4b = Ulceration or satellite nodules.
- T4c = T4a + T4b.
- T4d = Inflammatory carcinoma.

Lymph Nodes

- N0 = No lymph node metastases.
- N1 = Levels I, II moveable ipsilateral positive nodes in axilla.
- N1mi = Microscopic metastases, less than 1 mm in greatest dimension.
- N2a = Fixed levels I, II ipsilateral axillary nodes.
- N2b = Clinically detected nodes in the ipsilateral internal mammary chain without axillary nodal involvement.
- N3a = Metastases in ipsilateral infraclavicular nodes.
- N3b = Metastases in ipsilateral internal mammary chain and in axilla.
- N3c = Metastases in ipsilateral supraclavicular nodes.

Metastases

- M0 = No distant metastases.
- M1 = Distant metastases present.

Stages

- Stage 0 = Tis N0 M0.
- Stage IA = T1 N0 M0.
- Stage IB = T0 N1mi M0 or T1 N1mi M0.
- Stage IIA = T0 N1 M0 or T1 N1 M0 or T2 N0 M0.
- Stage IIB = T2 N1 M0 or T3 N0 M0.
- Stage IIIA = T0 N2 M0 or T1 N2 M0 or T2 N2 M0 or T3 N1 M0 or
- T3 N1 M0 or T3 N2 M0.
- Stage IIIB = T4 N0 M0 or T4 N1 M0 or T4 N2 M0.
- Stage IIIC = Any T N3 M0.
- Stage IV = Ant T, Any N, M1.

While TNM (tumor size, node involvement, and metastasis status) staging has been important in the determination of prognosis, the genetic analysis of the tumors not only has led to more targeted therapies, but also has been utilized for prognosis.

Surgery

In recently diagnosed breast cancer, surgery is the mainstay of therapy in stages I, II, and T3N1M0 disease.[4] Contraindications to surgery are distant metastases although it has been suggested that there is a survival benefit for removal of the primary tumor in patients with distant metastases.[6] Breast conserving surgery ("lumpectomy") followed by radiation therapy (RT) rather than mastectomy allows a better cosmetic result without sacrificing survival since most deaths are not due to recurrence of the primary but due to metastases.[7] Recurrence at the primary site is more likely in patients who meet the following criteria:

- Young (<40 years old).
- Have the *BRCA1* or *BRCA2* gene mutation.
- Have the molecular subtype of the tumor.
- Have less than R0 resection, leaving either macroscopic or microscopic disease at the margin.

- Lack boost of radiation to the surgical site.
- No systemic adjuvant chemotherapy is utilized.[8,9]

Patients who wish to have breast conserving surgery but have larger tumors may undergo neoadjuvant chemotherapy to shrink the tumor. This strategy is most effective in patients having a single lesion, high-grade more aggressive, HER2-positive or triple-negative tumors.[10,11]

Chemotherapy

Patients with estrogen-receptor (ER) or progesterone-receptor (PR) positive tumors are usually treated with hormonal therapy such as tamoxifen for at least 5 years resulting in a 40% reduction in the annual recurrence rate and a 34% reduction in the annual death rate.[12] An aromatase inhibitor binds to the ER and prevents the conversion of androgens into estrogen. These drugs should be part of the chemotherapy regimen in postmenopausal women since premenopausal women will overcome the effects of the aromatase inhibitor by producing more ovarian estrogen.[13,14]

In patients whose tumor lacks the ER (ER negative), the PR (PR negative), and the HER2 receptor (HER2 negative), treatment with hormonal therapy or anti-HER2 therapy is ineffective. Chemotherapy with multiple cycles of cyclophosphamide and doxorubicin doublet therapy has historically been utilized. The introduction of taxanes, such as paclitaxel, has improved survival when it is utilized sequentially with the cyclophosphamide–doxorubicin regimen.[15]

Patients having a tumor that is HER2 positive should have trastuzumab added to their chemotherapy regimen.

Radiation Therapy

RT is an integral part of the management of both primary breast cancer and metastatic disease. If breast conserving surgery is performed, it is followed by a 50-Gy RT whole-breast irradiation or partial-breast irradiation and a 10- to 16-Gy boost given to the operative bed. The recurrence rate at both 5- and 10-year follow-up demonstrated a significant difference between those patients who received the boost and those who did not (6.2 vs. 10.2%, respectively).[16,17]

Prognosis

Local–regional recurrence occurs in 4 to 10% of patients at 10 years.[18] These recurrences are usually treated by excision followed by additional radiation if possible followed by chemotherapy of a different type than was used initially. The use of concurrent chemotherapy with radiation reduces the risk of further spread and improved survival particularly in ER-negative patients.[19] Death is usually the result of metastatic disease to brain or liver.

The Role of Interventional Radiology

The contribution of interventional radiology to the management of breast cancer is limited to placement of vascular access, treatment of bony and liver metastases, and management of chronic malignant pleural effusions. There is some evidence that some breast cancers may be treated with radiofrequency ablation instead of surgery if surgical therapy is not an option.[20]

References

1. Lakhani SR, Ellis IO, Schnitt SJ, et al. World Health Organization Classification of Tumours of the Breast. 4th ed. Lyon, France: IARC Press; 2012

2. Velculescu VE. Defining the blueprint of the cancer genome. Carcinogenesis 2008;29(6):1087–1091

3. Olopade OI, Grushko TA, Nanda R, Huo D. Advances in breast cancer: pathways to personalized medicine. Clin Cancer Res 2008;14(24):7988–7999

4. DeVita VT, Lawrence TS, Rosenberg SA. Cancer: Principles and Practice of Oncology. Philadelphia, PA: Wolters Kluwer; 2015

5. Edge SB, Byrd DR, Compton CC, eds. AJCC Cancer Staging Manual. 7th ed. New York, NY: Springer; 2010

6. Rapiti E, Verkooijen HM, Vlastos G, et al. Complete excision of primary breast tumor improves survival of patients with metastatic breast cancer at diagnosis. J Clin Oncol 2006;24(18):2743–2749

7. Clarke M, Collins R, Darby S, et al; Early Breast Cancer Trialists' Collaborative Group (EBCTCG). Effects of radiotherapy and of differences in the extent of surgery for early breast cancer on local recurrence and 15-year survival: an overview of the randomised trials. Lancet 2005;366(9503):2087–2106

8. Arvold ND, Taghian AG, Niemierko A, et al. Age, breast cancer subtype approximation, and local recurrence after breast-conserving therapy. J Clin Oncol 2011;29(29):3885–3891

9. Lowery AJ, Kell MR, Glynn RW, Kerin MJ, Sweeney KJ. Locoregional recurrence after breast cancer surgery: a systematic review by receptor phenotype. Breast Cancer Res Treat 2012;133(3):831–841

10. Gianni L, Pienkowski T, Im YH, et al. Efficacy and safety of neoadjuvant pertuzumab and trastuzumab in women with locally advanced, inflammatory, or early HER2-positive breast cancer (NeoSphere): a randomised multicentre, open-label, phase 2 trial. Lancet Oncol 2012;13(1):25–32

11. Mauri D, Pavlidis N, Ioannidis JP. Neoadjuvant versus adjuvant systemic treatment in breast cancer: a meta-analysis. J Natl Cancer Inst 2005;97(3):188–194

12. Davies C, Pan H, Godwin J, et al; Adjuvant Tamoxifen: Longer Against Shorter (ATLAS) Collaborative Group. Long-term effects of continuing adjuvant tamoxifen to 10 years versus stopping at 5 years after diagnosis of oestrogen receptor-positive breast cancer: ATLAS, a randomised trial. Lancet 2013;381(9869):805–816

13. Goss PE, Ingle JN, Pritchard KI, et al. Exemestane versus anastrozole in postmenopausal women with early breast cancer: NCIC CTG MA.27--a randomized controlled phase III trial. J Clin Oncol 2013;31(11):1398–1404

14. Burstein HJ, Prestrud AA, Seidenfeld J, et al; American Society of Clinical Oncology. American Society of Clinical Oncology clinical practice guideline: update on adjuvant endocrine therapy for women with hormone receptor-positive breast cancer. J Clin Oncol 2010;28(23):3784–3796

15. Fisher B, Jeong JH, Anderson S, Wolmark N. Treatment of axillary lymph node-negative, estrogen receptor-negative breast cancer: updated findings from National Surgical Adjuvant Breast and Bowel Project clinical trials. J Natl Cancer Inst 2004;96(24):1823–1831

16. Bartelink H, Horiot JC, Poortmans PM, et al. Impact of a higher radiation dose on local control and survival in breast-conserving therapy of early breast cancer: 10-year results of the randomized boost versus no boost EORTC 22881-10882 trial. J Clin Oncol 2007;25(22):3259–3265

17. Daugherty EC, Daugherty MR, Bogart JA, Shapiro A. Adjuvant radiation improves survival in older women following breast-conserving surgery for estrogen receptor-negative breast cancer. Clin Breast Cancer 2016;16(6):500–506.e2

18. Anderson SJ, Wapnir I, Dignam JJ, et al. Prognosis after ipsilateral breast tumor recurrence and locoregional recurrences in patients treated by breast-conserving therapy in five National Surgical Adjuvant Breast and Bowel Project protocols of node-negative breast cancer. J Clin Oncol 2009;27(15):2466–2473

19. Aebi S, Gelber S, Lang I, et al. Chemotherapy prolongs survival for isolated local or regional recurrence of breast cancer: the CALOR trial (chemotherapy as adjuvant for locally recurrent breast cancer; IBCSG 27–02, NSABP B-37, BIG 1–02). Cancer Res 2012;72(24):S3–2

20. Barral M, Auperin A, Hakime A, et al. Percutaneous thermal ablation of breast cancer metastases in oligometastatic patients. Cardiovasc Intervent Radiol 2016;39(6):885–893

17 Gynecologic Tumors

Douglas M. Coldwell

Endometrial Cancer

Epidemiology

Endometrial cancer is the most common gynecologic malignancy with uterine sarcomas and is very rare (3%). The etiology is thought to be the chronic stimulation of the endometrium by estrogen, unopposed by progesterone.

Risk Factors

Risk factors[1–4] of endometrial cancer include the following:

- Early menarche.
- Late menopause.
- Nulliparity.
- Morbid obesity.
- Non-insulin-dependent diabetes.
- Hypertension.
- Use of tamoxifen in postmenopausal breast cancer.
- Use of estrogen-only hormone replacement therapy.

Genetics

Lynch's syndrome due to faulty deoxyribonucleic acid (DNA) mismatch repair genes, autosomal dominant.[5]

Pathology

Endometrial hyperplasia is the precursor lesion for endometrioid adenocarcinoma, which is the most common (75%), and is graded by the amount of solid masses within tumor cells; the larger the solid masses, the higher the grade. Endometrial thickening can be seen on transvaginal ultrasound or magnetic resonance imaging.[6,7]

Serous carcinoma (uterine papillary serous cancer) represents about 10% of endometrial carcinoma and is aggressive with early spread to lymph nodes and peritoneum.[8]

Tumor Syndromes

Lynch's syndrome (hereditary nonpolyposis colorectal cancer) can be associated with about 5% of endometrial cancer, presents 40–60% risk of endometrial cancer, and results in lower mean age of onset than the general population.

Staging

The International Federation of Gynecology and Obstetrics Staging system[9] is used:

- Stage I: Tumor confined to body of the uterus.
  – IA: Less than half of the myometrium invaded.
  – IB: More than half of the myometrium invaded.
- Stage II: Invades cervical stroma but does not extend beyond uterus.
- Stage III: Locoregional spread of tumor.
- Stage IV: Invades bladder or bowel or has distant metastases.

Treatment

Treatment followed for different stages of endometrial cancer are as follows:

- Stages I–II: Simple hysterectomy/bilateral salpingo-oophorectomy (BSO).
  About 5% may have adnexal involvement.[10]
  If the patient is younger than 50 years, synchronous ovarian cancer may occur in 9% of cases. Laparoscopic hysterectomy has fewer postoperative adverse events with the same overall survival as with transabdominal hysterectomy. Radiation therapy (RT) with intravaginal brachytherapy is only indicated in patients older than 60 years with lymphovascular invasion in stage IA, grade 1 or 2. In higher grades, RT is indicated since vaginal recurrence may be as high as 14%.[11] Adjuvant chemotherapy is not usually used.
- Stage III: Heterogenous group of patients usually treated with chemoradiation with 50 Gy of intensity-modulated radiation therapy (IMRT) coupled with cisplatin (50 mg/m^2), then four courses

of paclitaxel/carboplatin. This regimen results in a 5-year disease-free survival of 88% and an overall survival at 5 years of 97%.[12]

- Stage IV: Incurable disease; however, the regimen of paclitaxel, cisplatin, and doxorubicin results in a 57% response rate, progression-free survival of 8.3 months, overall survival of 15 months.[13] Antiangiogenic agents, mTOR (mammalian target of rapamycin) inhibitors, anti-EGFR (anti-epidermal growth factor receptor) agents and numerous single-agent chemotherapy trials are ongoing for second-line chemotherapy.

Role for Interventional Radiology

Since this cancer may invade the bladder, renal obstruction and hydro-nephrosis are a possibility and are treated with percutaneous nephrostomy and ureteral stents. These tumors may also invade and cause hemorrhage, which can be treated with embolotherapy. Chemotherapy should not be utilized as this tumor is likely being treated with chemo-therapeutic agents that are nephrotoxic (such as cisplatin) and their addition does nothing to assist in the shrinkage of the tumor beyond the embolic effect. Particles that are approximately 100 µ in diameter are preferred since it is unlikely that they will result in necrosis, only isch-emia. Larger particles will produce collateral vessels almost immediately and will likely result in recurrent hemorrhage.

Cervical and Vaginal Cancer

Epidemiology

Both cervical and vaginal cancers are likely to have similar origins. About 60 to 65% of vaginal cancers are positive for human papillomavirus (HPV) infection and 99% of cervical cancers.[14]

Most vaginal cancers occur in elderly women over the age of 60 years.[15] Clear cell carcinoma is associated with maternal diethylstilbes-trol (DES) use and is present in women younger than 40 years.[16]

Over half of vaginal cancers occur in the superior one-third of the vagina and may directly invade the bladder, urethra, or rectum or have nodal spread at presentation (14%).[17]

Genetics

HPV is integrated into tumor DNA in the most aggressive tumors.

Pathology

About 80 to 90% of both vaginal and cervical cancers are squamous cell carcinomas with 5 to 10% being adenocarcinomas with a poorer prognosis.[18]

Staging of Vaginal Cancer

Staging of vaginal cancer[2] and treatment methods are as follows:

- Stage 0: Carcinoma in situ.
  Treatment: Laser ablation.

- Stage I : Limited to the vaginal wall.
  Treatment: RT with combination of external beam and brachytherapy of 40 to 50 Gy to pelvic nodes and 70 to 75 Gy to the tumor. Five-year survival rate is 75 to 95%.[19]

- Stage II: Involves subvaginal tissues but does not extend to pelvic wall.
  Treatment: Brachytherapy to the primary tumor with IMRT to the pelvic nodes. Survival rates of 67% are seen.[20] Radical surgery with radical vaginectomy or pelvic exenteration in patients with recurrent disease after radiation.

- Stage III : Extends to pelvic wall.
  Treatment: Brachytherapy with external beam to nodes. Five-year survival rate is 30 to 60%.

- Stage IV: Extends beyond true pelvis or invaded adjacent structures.

- Stage IVA: Extends beyond pelvis by direct extension or invades adjacent structures.
  Treatment: RT with brachytherapy and external beam to nodes. Five-year survival is 15 to 40%.

- Stage IVB: Spread to distant organs.

Staging for Cervical Cancer

Staging of cervical cancer[9] and treatment methods are as follows:

- Stage I: Confined to the cervix.

- Stage IA: Invasive carcinoma that can only be diagnosed by microscopy with deepest invasion less than 5 mm.

Treatment for I/IA: Therapeutic conization with negative margins or, if positive margins, added brachytherapy has a 95% rate of cure.[21]

- Stage IB: Clinically visible lesions limited to the cervix.

- Stage II: Invades beyond uterus but not to pelvic wall or to the inferior third of the vagina.
  Treatment for stages IB/II: Brachytherapy combined with external beam RT or radical hysterectomy and pelvic lymphadenectomy. Equivalent survival of 80 to 90% at 5 years.[22]

- Stage III: Extends to the pelvic wall or involves inferior third of the vagina or causes hydronephrosis

- Stage IV: Extends beyond true pelvis or involves bladder or rectum.

- Stage IVA: Involves adjacent organs.
  Treatment for stages II/III/IVA: Combination of external beam RT, usually IMRT, and brachytherapy. Five-year survival rates of 65 to 75%, 35 to 50%, and 15 to 20% for stages II, III, and IVA, respectively.[23,24]

- Stage IVB: Distant metastases.
  Treatment: Incurable. Doublet with carboplatin and paclitaxel used for symptomatic therapy for either stage IVB or recurrent. Survival is only a few months.[25]

Prognostic Factors

- Size of tumor: If greater than 4 cm in diameter, prognosis is worse than stage would predict.
- Lymph node metastases: Most important prognostic factor; survival is approximately halved with the presence of nodal metastases.
- Lymphovascular invasion or parametrial invasion has a poorer prognosis.
- Strong inflammatory response is a predictor of good response to therapy.
- Adenocarcinomas have a poorer prognosis.
- Anemia is prognostic for locoregional recurrence.

Role for Interventional Radiology

This tumor is much like the previously discussed gynecologic cancers in that hydronephrosis and hemorrhage are the primary symptoms that lead the patient to present to interventional radiology (IR). Percutaneous biopsy of these tumors is not suggested as there may be seeding of the needle track.

Ovarian Cancer

Since ovarian cancer is indolent until it presents as peritoneal carcinomatosis, there is no real role for IR procedures, and discussion of this entity will not be pursued.

References

1. McPherson CP, Sellers TA, Potter JD, Bostick RM, Folsom AR. Reproductive factors and risk of endometrial cancer. The Iowa Women's Health Study. Am J Epidemiol 1996;143(12):1195–1202

2. Zucchetto A, Serraino D, Polesel J, et al. Hormone-related factors and gynecological conditions in relation to endometrial cancer risk. Eur J Cancer Prev 2009;18(4):316–321

3. Dossus L, Allen N, Kaaks R, et al. Reproductive risk factors and endometrial cancer: the European Prospective Investigation into Cancer and Nutrition. Int J Cancer 2010;127(2):442–451

4. Saltzman BS, Doherty JA, Hill DA, et al. Diabetes and endometrial cancer: an evaluation of the modifying effects of other known risk factors. Am J Epidemiol 2008;167(5):607–614

5. Hampel H, Frankel W, Panescu J, et al. Screening for Lynch syndrome (hereditary nonpolyposis colorectal cancer) among endometrial cancer patients. Cancer Res 2006;66(15):7810–7817

6. Bell DJ, Pannu HK. Radiological assessment of gynecologic malignancies. Obstet Gynecol Clin North Am 2011;38(1):45–68, vii

7. Frei KA, Kinkel K, Bonél HM, Lu Y, Zaloudek C, Hricak H. Prediction of deep myometrial invasion in patients with endometrial cancer: clinical utility of contrast-enhanced MR imaging-a meta-analysis and Bayesian analysis. Radiology 2000;216(2):444–449

8. Cirisano FD Jr, Robboy SJ, Dodge RK, et al. Epidemiologic and surgicopathologic findings of papillary serous and clear cell endometrial cancers when compared to endometrioid carcinoma. Gynecol Oncol 1999;74(3):385–394

9. Pecorelli S. Revised FIGO staging for carcinoma of the vulva, cervix, and endometrium. Int J Gynaecol Obstet 2009;105(2):103–104

10. Creasman WT, Morrow CP, Bundy BN, Homesley HD, Graham JE, Heller PB. Surgical pathologic spread patterns of endometrial cancer. A Gynecologic Oncology Group Study. Cancer 1987; 60(8, Suppl):2035–2041

11. Sorbe B, Nordström B, Mäenpää J, et al. Intravaginal brachytherapy in FIGO stage I low-risk endometrial cancer: a controlled randomized study. Int J Gynecol Cancer 2009;19(5):873–878

12. Shih KK, Milgrom SA, Abu-Rustum NR, et al. Postoperative pelvic intensity-modulated radiotherapy in high risk endometrial cancer. Gynecol Oncol 2013;128(3):535–539

13. Fleming GF, Brunetto VL, Cella D, et al. Phase III trial of doxorubicin plus cisplatin with or without paclitaxel plus filgrastim in advanced endometrial carcinoma: a Gynecologic Oncology Group Study. J Clin Oncol 2004;22(11):2159–2166

14. International Agency for Research on Cancer (IARC). Monographs on the Evaluation of Carcinogenic Risks to Humans. Hu\man Papillomaviruses. Vol 64. Lyon, France: IARC; 1995

15. Shepherd J, Sideri M, Benedet J, et al. Carcinoma of the vagina. J Epidemiol Biostat 1998;3:103–109</jrn>

16. Hoover RN, Hyer M, Pfeiffer RM, et al. Adverse health outcomes in women exposed in utero to diethylstilbestrol. N Engl J Med 2011;365(14):1304–1314

17. Kirkbride P, Fyles A, Rawlings GA, et al. Carcinoma of the vagina: -experience at the Princess Margaret Hospital (1974-1989). Gynecol Oncol 1995;56(3):435–443

18. Frank SJ, Deavers MT, Jhingran A, Bodurka DC, Eifel PJ. Primary adenocarcinoma of the vagina not associated with diethylstilbestrol (DES) exposure. Gynecol Oncol 2007;105(2):470–474

19. Frank SJ, Jhingran A, Levenback C, Eifel PJ. Definitive radiation therapy for squamous cell carcinoma of the vagina. Int J Radiat Oncol Biol Phys 2005;62(1):138–147

20. Perez CA, Grigsby PW, Garipagaoglu M, Mutch DG, Lockett MA. Factors affecting long-term outcome of irradiation in carcinoma of the vagina. Int J Radiat Oncol Biol Phys 1999;44(1):37–45

21. Grigsby PW, Perez CA. Radiotherapy alone for medically inoperable carcinoma of the cervix: stage IA and carcinoma in situ. Int J Radiat Oncol Biol Phys 1991;21(2):375–378

22. Rotman M, Sedlis A, Piedmonte MR, et al. A phase III randomized trial of postoperative pelvic irradiation in Stage IB cervical carcinoma with poor prognostic features: follow-up of a gynecologic oncology group study. Int J Radiat Oncol Biol Phys 2006;65(1):169–176

23. Eifel PJ, Jhingran A, Levenback CF, Tucker S. Predictive value of a proposed subclassification of stages I and II cervical cancer based on clinical tumor diameter. Int J Gynecol Cancer 2009;19(1):2–7

24. Logsdon MD, Eifel PJ. Figo IIIB squamous cell carcinoma of the cervix: an analysis of prognostic factors emphasizing the balance between external beam and intracavitary radiation therapy. Int J Radiat Oncol Biol Phys 1999;43(4):763–775

25. Kitagawa R, Katsumata N, Ando M, et al. A multi-institutional phase II trial of paclitaxel and carboplatin in the treatment of advanced or recurrent cervical cancer. Gynecol Oncol 2012;125(2):307–311

18 Clinical Trials and Interventional Oncology

Douglas M. Coldwell

Introduction

To become integrated with most medical oncology groups, a good understanding of clinical trials is necessary, since interventional radiology (IR) is likely to be a key player in the trial, whether it is via obtaining a biopsy, injecting a lesion, or participating in novel therapeutic options. Most medical oncologists, and particularly those associated with universities, are very enthusiastic participants in these trials. It attracts patients to the center and allows both academic and private practices to contribute to research. The multicenter groups such as the Southwest Oncology Group (SWOG), the Cancer and Leukemia Group – B (CALGB), or the Radiation Therapy Oncology Group (RTOG) usually coordinate these activities. It is highly suggested that any IR participation in a clinical trial should entitle the IR to be listed as either a co-investigator or key personnel depending on the level of involvement so that the IR may receive the appropriate level of recognition for their contribution. To perform research under a national institute of health or other government-funded grant, any physician or researcher needs to be registered with the Department of Health and Human Services (DHHS) by completing Form 1571 obtained from the DHHS website.[1]

Drug versus Device Trial

The new treatment must first be determined to be either a drug or a device or a combination treatment. There are separate pathways for a drug or device but a combination therapy, for example, chemotherapy combined with a radiation treatment, must be assigned to a particular center. The device pathway is through the Center for Devices and Radiologic Health (CDRH), while the drug pathway is through the Center for Drug Evaluation and Research (CDER). CDER also oversees the following types of biological therapies:

- Monoclonal antibodies for in vivo use.
- Proteins intended for therapeutic use, including cytokines (e.g., interferons), enzymes (e.g., thrombolytics), and other novel proteins, except for those that are specifically assigned to CBER (e.g., vaccines and blood products). This category includes therapeutic proteins derived from plants, animals, or microorganisms, and recombinant versions of these products.
- Immunomodulators (nonvaccine and nonallergenic products intended to treat disease by inhibiting or modifying a pre-existing immune response).
- Growth factors, cytokines, and monoclonal antibodies intended to mobilize, stimulate, decrease, or otherwise alter the production of hematopoietic cells in vivo.

Other biologics go through the Center for Biologic Evaluation and Research (CBER) and include the following:

- Cellular products, including products composed of human, bacterial, or animal cells (such as pancreatic islet cells for transplantation), or from physical parts of those cells (such as whole cells, cell fragments, or other components intended for use as preventative or therapeutic vaccines).
- Gene therapy products. Human gene therapy/gene transfer is the administration of nucleic acids, viruses, or genetically engineered microorganisms that mediate their effect by transcription and/or translation of the transferred genetic material, and/or by integrating into the host genome. Cells may be modified in these ways ex vivo for subsequent administration to the recipient, or altered in vivo by gene therapy products administered directly to the recipient.
- Vaccines (products intended to induce or increase an antigen-specific immune response for prophylactic or therapeutic immunization, regardless of the composition or method of manufacture).
- Allergenic extracts used for the diagnosis and treatment of allergic diseases and allergen patch tests.
- Antitoxins, antivenins, and venoms.
- Blood, blood components, plasma-derived products (e.g., albumin, immunoglobulins, clotting factors, fibrin sealants, proteinase inhibitors), including recombinant and transgenic versions of plasma derivatives (e.g., clotting factors), blood substitutes, plasma volume expanders, human or animal polyclonal antibody preparations including radiolabeled or conjugated forms, and certain fibrinolytics such as plasma-derived plasmin, and red cell reagents.

A combination product, as defined in 21 CFR § 3.2(e), is a product comprised of any combination of a drug and a device; a biological product and a device; a drug and a biological product; or a drug, a device, and a biological product. The regulatory pathway for these will be assigned to the center for which the primary mode of action is determined. For instance, drug-eluting stents may go through either CDER or CDRH, but the primary mode of action is the stent so it went through CDRH. The Office of Combination Products at the Food and Drug Administration (FDA) makes this determination. Once the pathway is defined, a trial needs to be designed. For FDA approval, an initial trial is put together and discussed with the FDA before it is instituted so that any comments the FDA makes can be considered.

Trial Phases

Trials are classified into five phases:

- Phase 0: Exploratory study involving very limited human exposure to the drug with no therapeutic or diagnostic goals, for example, screening studies or microdose studies.
- Phase 1: Studies that are conducted with either healthy volunteers or terminally ill patients and that emphasize safety. The goal is to find out what the drug's most frequent and serious adverse events are and, often, how the drug is metabolized and excreted. For device studies, the particular device is also used in these patients to determine the most common complications and their frequency.
- Phase 2: Studies that gather preliminary data on effectiveness, whether the drug or device actually works in people who have a particular disease or condition. Safety continues to be evaluated and short-term adverse events are studied.
- Phase 1/2: Studies that combine the elements of determination of both safety and efficacy.
- Phase 3: Larger studies that gather more information about safety and efficacy by varying dosage, use in different populations, and using the drug in combination with other drugs. For devices, this is a large study that uses the device with standard of care therapy and compares the results to standard of care therapy alone. This study is usually referred to as the "pivotal" study that is used for premarket approval by the FDA.
- Phase 2/3: Studies that combine the elements of beginning to determine if the drug has efficacy and, if so, continuing to a larger trial.

- Phase 4: These studies occur after the FDA has approved the use of the drug or device. It may be a condition of approval to determine the effect on larger populations to determine the drug's optimal use, safety, and efficacy.

Types of Trials

These studies may be of four different types:

- Single group: A single group receives the drug or device treatment without a comparative group and uses historical controls. This is unusual for FDA approval trials.
- Parallel: Participants are assigned to one of two or more groups in parallel for the entire study. Each group receives one particular treatment and allows intergroup comparison. Care must be taken to insure that all groups have similar characteristics, for example, age, sex, gender, and disease state, so that the comparison can be valid.
- Crossover: Participants receive one of two interventions during the initial portion of the study and may have the second during the latter portion. The criteria for crossing over to the other intervention may be automatic or may be only after disease progression.
- Factorial: Two or more interventions, each alone and in combination, are evaluated in parallel in comparison to a control group. It should be noted that in oncology research "best supportive care" versus an intervention is not usually performed if there is a treatment available.

Other factors in the design of the study include if the participants will be "masked" or have knowledge of the intervention. An open study is one where no masking is utilized and all participants and physicians know the treatment that the patient underwent. A single-blind study is where one party, either the investigator or the participant, is unaware of the intervention. The use of placebo drugs allows the participants to be unaware if they are in the group not receiving the drug. Obviously, the use of a device is difficult to make the patients unaware of their participation. Sham surgeries or procedures have been performed but are increasingly difficult to justify due to their cost and risk to the patient. Double-blind studies are those where both parties, usually the investigator and the patient, are unaware of what drug is being utilized in their treatment. However, the caregiver or the outcome assessor can also be blinded to the treatment so as not to bias their judgment of the effectiveness if no quantifiable outcome can be obtained, for example, size of tumor as measured on computed tomography.

Studies must also consider the allocation of participants. The study may be randomized so that participants are assigned to intervention groups by chance, for example, if their medical record number is odd or even, or by a table of randomization generated for the study. Nonrandomized trials are those where the participants are expressly assigned to intervention groups, such as by their physician choice.

Study Endpoints

Study classification or endpoint determination is the type of primary outcome that the protocol is designed to evaluate. These include the following:

- Safety: if the drug is safe under the conditions of proposed use.
- Efficacy: measures the intervention's influence on a disease.
- Safety/efficacy: measures both safety and efficacy.
- Bioequivalence: compares generic and brand name drugs.
- Bioavailability: the rate and extent that a drug is absorbed and available to the treatment site.
- Pharmacokinetics: the action of the drug in the body over a period of time including the process of absorption, distribution and localization in tissues. Action of the *body on the drug.*
- Pharmacodynamics: action of drugs in living systems. Action of the *drug on the body*.

The enrollment or number of participants necessary to determine the statistical significance of the action of the drug or device is determined by how great is the anticipated response to treatment over and above the current levels of treatment response. If the anticipated response is only slight, a greater number of participants will be required to obtain a statistically significant response as opposed to one where the current therapy response is low and the anticipated response is great.

Prospective Studies

These protocols, which are generally for FDA approvals, are usually prospective. In other words, beginning today with the enrollment, the participants are observed and their response noted. In rare diseases, a historical control may sometimes be substituted for a control group of the current therapy. The observational study model utilized may be the following:

- Cohort: group of individuals, initially defined and composed with common characteristics (e.g., disease stage, treatment received, age) and followed over a given time period after receiving a particular intervention.

- Case control: a group of individuals with specific characteristics compared with groups with different characteristics but otherwise similar.
- Case only: a single group of individuals with specific characteristics.
- Case crossover: characteristics of case immediately prior to disease onset (called the "hazard period") compared with characteristics of the same case at a prior time (called the "control period").

A biostatistician is of invaluable assistance when designing a study as they are intimately familiar with the statistics necessary to analyze a study but must have the clinical input from the study investigators to successfully design a workable study that is successful. A well-designed study that does not enroll patients due to unnecessary limits placed on the patient, for example, they must receive their chemotherapy at the same clinic where the study is being held even though they may have to drive an excessive distance, would not be successful. A study that enrolls patients and is well executed must be performed in a reasonable time period or the results will not be significant as the advances in oncologic therapy are moving reasonably quickly. A study comparing a new device with and without "old" chemotherapy is of no use in obtaining the medical oncology community's approval and use.

A note must also be made on the types of FDA device approvals obtained. A Humanitarian Device Exemption (HDE) approval is one where the new device is likely to be effective and unlikely to be harmful to patients based on work performed in laboratory animals. This allows a company to sell the device for a particular purpose, for example, to treat hepatocellular carcinoma, only so that the company can garner the proceeds to perform a full-fledged phase 3 pivotal trial to determine its effectiveness and safety. Usually these approvals last for 3 to 5 years; then the FDA will ask the company to perform the pivotal trial. Premarket approval (PMA) is the approval earned by companies whose devices are proven effective and safe in the phase 3 pivotal trial. These devices, while approved for a particular use, may be used "off label" on the physician's discretion to treat other diseases not on the approved list for the particular device. The physician then assumes the liability for the use of the device. Finally, a 510(k) approval is that given to a device when a "predicate" device or one that is similar to the new device has already been given PMA approval and the new device may be similar but with new features that do not substantially change the performance of the device. This is why there are numerous approved subcutaneous ports, tunneled dialysis catheters, etc., present in the market.[1]

Additionally, membership in the Association of Clinical Research Professionals can be of great help.[2] Being designated as a Certified Physician Investigator (CPI) also gives credibility to the IR's competency in performing clinical trials. To become a CPI requires passing an examination that covers the following:

- Scientific concepts and research design.
- Ethical and participant safety considerations.
- Product development and regulation.
- Clinical trial operations (GCPs).
- Study and site management.
- Data management and informatics.

While this may seem daunting, the rewards are that any trials in which the IR participates can be assured to be well designed and run.

References

1. FDA web site. www.FDA.gov. Accessed November 22, 2016
2. Association of Clinical Research Professionals website. www.acrpnet.org Accessed November 22, 2016

19 Building an Interventional Oncology Practice

Douglas M. Coldwell

Like much in medicine, new practices and procedures must have adequate clinical studies for background, an unmet need to be filled, or a new and better way to treat patients to become accepted. Interventional radiology has, for years, demonstrated to referring physicians that the endovascular, image-guided approach is preferable or adjunctive to many medical therapies and certainly less invasive than surgery. But given the lack of large clinical trials, level-1 evidence, and already established referral patterns, how does an interventional oncology (IO) practice grow and thrive? Actually it sounds very straightforward, but the execution is difficult.

First, get yourself a copy of a general medical oncology text and start studying. This information has not been taught to radiologists in residency or in medical school. Look at the treatment regimens, their response rates, and the survival rate. Know the common diseases very well and understand where minimally invasive image-guided techniques may benefit the patient. Two other books would also be helpful: one on molecular biology and the other on immunology. Much of the future of cancer therapy is based on understanding the molecular biology and genetics of the tumor and designing a drug or treatment to exploit it. Immunology has recently come to the field of oncology through the use of immune checkpoint inhibitors and the understanding of the immunology of the tumor.

Second, learn "onc-speak," or talk like an oncologist. There are several terms that they use that are not found outside of the field:

- Doublet: A combination of two chemotherapy agents; singlets are rarely used, but triplets are often used.
- Dose dense chemotherapy: Chemotherapy regimen that has less time between agents than standard chemotherapy.
- OS: Overall survival or the time from diagnosis of the cancer until death
- PFS: Progression-free survival—the time from the initiation of a therapy until the disease progresses. There can be a PFS for the liver, with liver-directed therapy and an overall PFS for spread beyond the liver, for example, lymph nodes.
- SOC: Standard of care.

- SD: Stable disease—no change in the index lesion(s) on cross-sectional imaging in a particular time period.
- PD: Progressive disease—increase in the size of the index lesion as determined by the measuring system employed, for example, mRECIST (modified response evaluation criteria in solid tumors). It is usually greater than a 25% increase in size of the lesion's greatest diameter.
- PR: Partial response—less than a 25% increase in size of the lesion's greatest diameter.
- CR: Complete response or eradication of the imaged disease, not necessarily cure since the patient must be followed for 3 to 5 years for that determination.
- RR: Response rate—the sum of the SD and CR and PR.
- QoL: Quality of life as measured by commonly accepted tools such as the SF-86, but there are quite specific measures for various tumors.
- ALBI: This score is a combination of the albumin and bilirubin levels by a specific formula that removes the qualitative judgment from the Childs–Pugh cirrhosis levels and is very prognostic.
- Cytoreductive therapy: Any therapy that locally removes tumors, for example, RFA (radiofrequency ablation) so that the grams of chemotherapy applied per gram of tumor is increased.
- Immuno-oncologic therapy: The use of the patient's own immune system to fight the tumor. For example, the use of PD-1 immune check point inhibitors that prevent this protein on the outside of T-cells from binding with its ligand, PD-L1. When PD-1 binds with PD-L1, the T-cell is prevented from attacking any cells, in this case tumor cells. There are also immune checkpoint inhibitors that bind to the ligand and perform the same function.

Third, attend every multidisciplinary tumor board available at your hospital, but do NOT under any circumstance show the imaging studies. If you show the imaging, you will be identified with "them," the non-treating physicians, making the task of building a practice much more difficult. Depending on the size of the group, sending two radiologists to every tumor board sounds excessive, but given the downstream increase in referred studies due to the IO practice, it is well worth it. The list of patients and their tumors is usually published a few days in advance, which will allow review of the disease, the pathology, and then think about the potential for IO intervention. If you think that the patient to be discussed would benefit from IO, look up the pertinent references on PubMed or in JVIR (Journal of Vascular and Interventional Radiology) and know the results so that when another clinician questions your outcomes, you will be informed. Take copies of the articles to the tumor board if it is a controversial case. Sit with the surgeons and medical oncologists and get to know them on a personal basis. Do not be afraid to speak during the discussion as it will show your knowledge (or lack thereof, so be careful!) and weigh in on whether a patient should have IO intervention.

Fourth, if you can arrange to get clinic space in the same physical space as the medical oncologists, you will manage to see them at least once a week in a setting where the IO is treating patients just like the medical oncologist. In such a setting, it is only natural for a bond to form between the medical oncologist and the IO so that the IO is seen as a partner not just as a doer of procedures. It makes it very convenient then for the medical oncologist to immediately refer the patient to the IO and start the referral process. An alternative is to have the oncologist call you to come to their clinic for a consultation, particularly if the patient lives far away, if it is inconvenient for the patient to return for a clinic appointment with the IO. Remember an effort to make it easy for the oncologist (e.g., one phone call) and easy for the patient to see you will result in an increase in the oncologic volume. Demonstrations that you are flexible enough to make the patient a priority go a long way to getting the oncologist to trust you.

Fifth, see ALL patients for therapy in the clinic first. After all, referring a patient to surgery will result in a clinic appointment and not an operating room date. This will allow the independent evaluation of the patient by the IO team and perhaps some refinement of the treatment plan.

Sixth, the cancer center is usually a semiseparate entity that has its own faculty or members. After regular attendance at the tumor boards, it will be only natural to become a faculty/member of the cancer center.

Seventh, if there is enough available manpower in IR, get and use your admitting privileges. This way the IO can take care of the patient without burdening the medical oncology service. And do not hesitate to consult specialists.

Eighth, join the American Society of Clinical Oncologists. Yes, there are nonmedical oncologist members. Display your membership certificate in your clinic or office. This also gives you a subscription to the Journal of Clinical Oncology, the place to find out what is going on in your major referrer's community and what the direction of therapy is for a particular disease so you can discuss it intelligently. It also shows your commitment to oncology and your dedication to keeping current.

Ninth, read a book on sales and marketing. Yes, that's right. The IO is selling his/her abilities and therapies to the medical oncologist. Recognize that they are the customer and go out and see them in their office, in clinic, on the oncology floor; get in their face and sell.

There is an old adage about consulting physicians: the 3As.

- Available. You need to be able to be easily contacted by referring physicians so that you get the cases. Hire the best people available to answer the telephones since they are the "face" of your practice. They need to know your policies on scheduling, holding anticoagulants, referring physicians getting the report, admissions, etc. The best practice is to have a "one call" referral: if the medical oncologist can get the patient in to see the IO in one call, a clinic appointment made with the patient, and then therapy discussed. Before the therapy is instituted, make a call or, preferably, send a written plan to the oncologist to outline the therapy discussed. One of the two biggest complaints about referring patients to the IO is the lack of communication so that the referring physician is apprised of what is going on. They do not want to feel left out of the loop. Send them the treatment plan, all dictations, and a plan for follow-up. The other complaint is that no adequate follow-up plans are made. If follow-up is due in 2 weeks by telephone call or clinic visit, it needs to be recorded in the chart and the referring oncologist notified of both the plan and the results of the call.
- Affable. Be nice. You do not need to be obsequious as you only get the respect you demand. Be firm and stick to your boundaries. There is a fine line between demanding respect and being arrogant. Be sure that you are on the right side of that line.
- Able. You need to know what you are talking about and be able to deliver. The absolute worst thing to do is to overpromise and underdeliver. In the process of building any practice, but specifically an IO one, prove your abilities in the easy cases building up to the more difficult ones. You may want the difficult ones immediately, but if there is a complication you won't have a reservoir of goodwill on which to draw. Nothing will kill an IO practice faster than having a serious complication on an early case. This is true for new physicians at any hospital. You may be experienced, but if you are a newcomer, you still have to prove your abilities to a new audience.

This undoubtedly sounds like a lot of work—it is! But if you want a quality IO practice, follow the above guidelines and words of wisdom because THEY WORK. It is not instantaneous, but with patience and persistence, it pays off.

Index

Note: Page numbers followed by *f* and *t* indicate figures and tables, respectively.

A

abdominal pain management, 76–81, 78*f*, 80–86*f*
Abraxane (paclitaxel), 99
adriamycin (doxorubicin), 92
afatinib, 144
aflibercept, 108
ALBI score, 207
allopurinol, 88
American College of Radiology (ACR), 17, 18
American Society for Therapeutic Radiology and Oncology (ASTRO), 17–18
amifostine, 88
androgen deprivation therapy, 178, 179
angioplasty, 63–66, 64–66*f*
antiepidermal growth factor receptors, 108
Association of Clinical Research Professionals, 205
ATRX mutation, 117
Avastin (bevacizumab), 2*t*, 89, 108, 164

B

balloon occlusion catheter, 50
BCNU (carmustine), 89
benign prostatic hyperplasia, 180–181
beta-catenin mutation, 126
bevacizumab (Avastin), 2*t*, 89, 108, 164
biliary drainage, percutaneous, 61–62, 63–64*f*
biopsy, image-guided, 33–36, 35*f*
biostatisticians, 204
Birt–Hogg–Dubé syndrome, 161
bladder cancer staging, 169–170
bleeding tumors, 48, 49*f*
bleomycin, 89
bony metastatic disease
  contraindications, 72
  external beam radiation therapy, 73

lung cancer (non–small cell), 151
prostate cancer, 179, 181–182
radiofrequency ablation, 73–76, 74–75*f*
vertebral augmentation, 72–76, 74–75*f*, 77*f*
brachytherapy
  principles, 19, 22–27
  prostate cancer, 178
BRAF mutation, 104
BRCA1, *BRCA2*, 185
breast cancer
  chemotherapy, 188
  epidemiology, 185
  genetics of, 185–186
  interventional radiology, 189
  pathology, 185
  prognosis, 189
  radiation therapy, 188
  recurrence, 189
  staging (TNM), 186–187
  surgery, 187–188

C

cabazitaxel, 179
capecitabine (Xeloda), 90
carboplatin, 99
carcinogenesis, 27
carcinoid tumor
  carcinoid syndrome, 123
  chemotherapy, 123
  diagnosis, 122
  epidemiology, 122
  locoregional therapies, 124
  pathology, 122
  staging, 122
  surgery, 123
carmustine (BCNU), 89
carotid blowout, 64–66, 67*f*
CDKN2A/p16 mutation, 113

celiac origin variants, 56, 56–57t
celiac plexus block, 69, 70f
Center for Devices and Radiologic Health
    (CDRH), 199–201
Center for Drug Evaluation and Research
    (CDER), 199–201
ceritinib, 144
Certified Physician Investigator (CPI) desig-
    nation, 205
cervical cancer, 193–196
cetuximab (Erbitux), 2t, 90, 108, 157
chemoembolization, 51–52, 53f
chemotherapy
    as adjuvant therapy, 4, 4t, 6
    agents (see specific agents by name)
    breast cancer, 188
    carcinoid tumor, 123
    cholangiocarcinoma, 134, 136
    colorectal cancer, 108
    combination, 103
    as concomitant therapy with radiation,
        4–5, 5t
    dose, schedule adjustments, 6
    dose dense, 206
    drug holidays, 6
    gallbladder cancer, 140
    head and neck tumors, 156–157
    hepatic arterial infusion, 61
    hepatocellular carcinoma, 129
    induction, maintenance regimens, 6
    lung cancer (non–small cell), 144, 149
    for palliation, 5–6, 7t
    pancreatic cancer, 115
    pancreatic neuroendocrine tumor, 117,
        119
    as primary therapy, 3, 4t
    prostate cancer, 179
    renal cell carcinoma, 164
    supportive/symptomatic measures, 6, 7t
    transitional cell cancer, 171
    urothelial cancers, 171
cholangiocarcinoma
    chemotherapy, 134, 136
    diagnosis, 133
    distal, staging, 137
    distal, treatment, 138
    genetics, 133
    locoregional therapy, 135
    palliation, 136–137
    pathology, 132
    perihilar, staging, 135–136
    perihilar, treatment, 136–137
    predisposing factors, 132
    prognosis, 134
    staging (TNM), 133–134
    surgery, 134
cholelithiasis. see gallbladder cancer
chronic cholelithiasis. see gallbladder cancer
cisplatin (Platinol), 79, 99, 157
clear cell carcinoma, 193
clinical trials
    ACRP membership, 205
    design of, 202–203
    drug vs. device, 199–201
    endpoints, 203
    FDA device approvals, 204
    overview, 199
    phases of, 201–202
    prospective studies, 203–205
    types of, 202–203
coil embolization, 48–52, 49f, 53f, 61
colorectal cancer
    chemotherapy, 108
    epidemiology, 104
    genetics of, 104
    prognosis, 107
    screening, 105–106
    staging (TNM), 106–107
    surgery, 107–108
    tumor syndromes, 105
consulting physicians, 208–209
Cowden's disease, 105, 162, 185
CR, 207
crizotinib, 3t, 144
crossover trials, 202
cryotherapy, 40–41
cyclophosphamide (Cytoxan), 90
cytoreductive therapy, 207

D

dacarbazine (DTIC), 91
daratumumab, 2t
daunorubicin, 91
DAXX mutation, 117
denosumab, 179

diarrhea treatment, 54*f*
dihydrotestosterone, 180
docetaxel (Taxotere), 91, 179
doublet, 206
doxorubicin (adriamycin), 92

E

EBRT. *see* external beam radiation therapy
EGFR mutation, 144, 168–169
embolization, preoperative, 82–83
embolotherapy, 48–52, 49*f*, 53*f*
endometrial cancer, 191–193
epidermitis, 27
epidural block, 72
epirubicin, 92
epoetin alfa (EPO, Procrit, Epogen), 92
Epogen, 92
Erbitux (cetuximab), 2*t*, 90, 108, 157
erlotinib (Tarceva), 3*t*, 93, 144
ethanol, 48–50
etoposide (VP-16), 93
external beam radiation therapy
    bony metastatic disease, 73
    lung cancer (non–small cell), 147
    principles, 19, 21–22, 24
    prostate cancer, 178–179

F

facial nerve block, 71–72
factorial trials, 202
familial adenomatous polyposis, 105
familial diffuse gastric cancer, 186
familial leiomyomatosis, 162
femoral block, 69–70
fibrolamellar hepatocellular carcinoma, 130
filgrastim (GCSF, Neupogen), 93
5-fluorouracil (5-FU), 94
510(k) approval, 204
floxuridine (FUDR), 94
FOLFIRINOX/FOLFOXIRI regimen, 103
FOLFIRI regimen, 103, 108
FOLFOX regimen, 103, 108
folinic acid (leucovorin), 97

G

gallbladder cancer
    chemotherapy, 140
    epidemiology, 138
    genetics, 139
    interventional radiology, 141
    pathology, 139
    prognosis, 141
    radiation therapy, 141
    staging (TNM), 139–140
    surgery, 140
Gardner's syndrome, 105
gastrointestinal tract neuroendocrine
       tumors. *see* carcinoid tumor
GCSF (filgrastim), 93
Gem/Abraxane regimen, 103
gemcitabine (Gemzar), 94
Gleevec (imatinib), 3*t*, 95
glossary, 206–207
glue, 50
gynecologic cancer, 79, 82*f*

H

head and neck tumors
    chemotherapy, 156–157
    epidemiology, 154
    genetics of, 154
    locoregional therapy, 158
    pain management, 79, 80*f*
    pathology, 154
    prognosis, 157, 159
    radiotherapy, 157
    staging (TNM), 154–155
    surgery, 156
hemorrhage, as biopsy complication, 34
hepatic arterial infusion, 61
hepatocellular carcinoma
    chemotherapy, 129
    epidemiology, 126
    fibrolamellar, 130
    pathology, genetics, 126
    prognosis, 127, 128
    radiofrequency ablation, 129
    staging (TNM), 127

surgery, 127–128
transplant, 128–129
HER2, 185
hereditary nonpolyposis colorectal cancer (HNPCC), 105
Hickman catheter (tunneled central line), 42–43*f*, 42–44, 45–46*f*
Humanitarian Device Exemption (HDE), 204
human papilloma virus (HPV), 154
Hunter, John, 11
hydrodissection, 37–38, 40*f*
hypervascular tumors, 79–81, 83–84*f*

I

idarubicin, 95
ifosfamide, 95
imaging, history of, 17
imatinib (Gleevec), 3*t*, 95
immuno-oncologic therapy, 207
implantable ports, 44–47
intensity-modulated radiation therapy, 178
interleukin-2 (IL-2), 96
interventional oncology practice, 206–209
interventional radiology
    angioplasty, 63–66, 64–66*f*
    biopsy, image-guided, 33–36, 35*f*
    breast cancer, 189
    gallbladder cancer, 141
    hepatic arterial infusion, 61
    implantable ports, 44–47
    lung cancer (non–small cell), 149–151
    overview, 33
    percutaneous biliary drainage, 61–62, 63–64*f*
    percutaneous nephrostomy, 66–68
    stenting, 63–66, 64–66*f*
    therapies, 48, 49*f*
    tumor ablation, 36–41, 38–40*f*
    venous access devices, 41–44, 42–43*f*, 45–46*f*
intrahepatic CCA. *see* cholangiocarcinoma
ipilimumab (Yervoy), 2, 2*t*, 96
irinotecan, 51–52, 96
irreversible electroporation (IRE), 41

K

Keytruda (pembrolizumab), 2, 2*t*, 100
KRAS mutation, 104, 113, 139, 144

L

leucovorin (folinic acid), 97
Li–Fraumeni syndrome, 185
liver
    metastases, pain management, 79–81, 83–84*f*
    radiotherapy effects on, 28–29
lung cancer (non–small cell)
    bony metastases disease, 151
    chemoradiation, 147–148
    chemotherapy, 144, 149
    epidemiology, 144
    external beam radiation therapy, 147
    genetics of, 144
    hemoptysis, 149–150
    interventional radiology, 149–151
    pain management, 150–151
    pathology, 144
    pleural effusions, malignant, 150
    prognosis, 147–148
    radiofrequency ablation, 151
    staging (TNM), 145–146
    surgery, 147–148
    SVC encroachment, 150
Lynch's syndrome, 105, 191, 192

M

medullary carcinoma, 161
MEK1 mutation, 144
MELD scores, 128
MEN1/MEN2a mutation, 117
methotrexate, 97
MET mutation, 144
microspheres, 25, 55–58
Milan criteria, 128–129
mitomycin C, 97
mitoxantrone, 98, 179
monoclonal antibodies, 2, 2–3*t*
mRECIST, 207
mucositis, 27

multilocular cystic RCC, 161
MVAC regimen, 103

N

Navelbine (vinorelbine), 103
nephrostomy, percutaneous, 66–68
Neupogen (filgrastim), 93
neuroendocrine tumors, gastrointestinal
    tract. *see* carcinoid tumor
neurofibromatosis type 1, 118
Nexavar (sorafenib), 3*t*, 58–59, 101, 129
nivolumab, 2
non–small cell lung cancer. *see* lung cancer
    (non–small cell)

O

observational study model, 203–204
occipital block, 72
octreotide (sandostatin), 98
Ohm's law, 181
ondansetron (Zofran), 98
osteosarcoma, 79
ovarian cancer, 196
oxaliplatin, 99

P

paclitaxel (Taxol, Abraxane), 99
pain management
    abdominal, due to mass effect, 76–81,
        78*f*, 80–86*f*
    bony metastatic disease (*see* bony meta-
        static disease)
    celiac plexus block, 69, 70*f*
    embolization, preoperative, 82–83
    epidural block, 72
    facial nerve block, 71–72
    femoral block, 69–70
    lung cancer (non–small cell), 150–151
    nerve blocks, 68
    occipital block, 72
    paracentesis/thoracentesis, 83–85
    pudendal block, 69, 71*f*
    splanchnic block, 69
    stellate ganglion block, 71
    vertebral augmentation, 72–76, 74–75*f*,
        77*f*

Pancoast tumors, 147
pancreatic cancer
    chemotherapy, 115
    diagnosis, 114
    epidemiology, 113
    genetics of, 113
    locoregional therapy, 115–116
    pathology, 113
    recurrence of, 115
    staging (TNM), 114
    surgery, 114–115
pancreatic neuroendocrine tumor
    chemotherapy, 117, 119
    epidemiology, 116
    genetics of, 117–118
    pathology, 116–117
    prognosis, 119–120
    staging (TNM), 118
    surgery, 119
    symptoms, 116
panitumumab (Vectibix), 99
paracentesis/thoracentesis, 83–85
particle size, 50–51
PD, 207
pembrolizumab (Keytruda), 2, 2*t*, 100
percutaneous biliary drainage, 61–62,
    63–64*f*
percutaneous nephrostomy, 66–68
peripherally inserted central catheters
    (PICCs), 46–47
Peutz–Jeghers syndrome, 105, 186
PFS (progression-free survival), 206
PIK3CA mutation, 117, 144
Platinol (cisplatin), 79, 99, 157
pneumothorax, 33, 34, 35*f*, 38*f*, 43
ports, implantable, 44–47
postembolization syndrome, 56, 58–59*f*, 76
PR, 207
practice, building, 206–209
premarket approval (PMA), 204
Procrit, 92
prostate cancer
    bony metastases, 179, 181–182
    chemotherapy, 179
    clinically localized disease, 177
    diagnosis, 176
    epidemiology, 175

external beam radiation therapy, 178–179
hyperplasia, prostate embolization, 180–181
locoregional therapy, 180
pain management, 179
pathology, 175
radiation therapy, 178–179
radiofrequency ablation, 181–182
staging (TNM), 176–177
surgery, 178
treatment, 177
PTEN mutation, 117
pudendal block, 69, 71*f*

Q

quality of life (QOL), 5–6

R

radiation hepatitis/RILD, 28, 29, 52–54
radiation oncology
absorbed dose estimation, 27–28
continuous low-dose, 19
governing bodies, 17–18
history of, 16–17
microspheres, 25, 55–58
MIRD, 28
normal tissues, effects in, 27–29
NTCP models, 28
overview, 16
physics of, 20–21
scope of practice, 18–19
3D modeling, 19, 20–21*f*
treatment approaches, 19, 20–21*f*
radiation pneumonitis, 27
radiation recall effect, 79, 80*f*
radical prostatectomy, 178
radiobiology, 23–29
radioembolization, 52–60, 54*f*, 56–57*t*, 58–59*f*
radioembolization-induced liver disease (REILD), 55
radiofrequency ablation
bony metastatic disease, 73–76, 74–75*f*
hepatocellular carcinoma, 129
local tumor therapy, 36–41, 38–40*f*
lung cancer (non–small cell), 151

prostate cancer, 181–182
renal cell carcinoma, 37, 40*f*, 50, 163
rectal cancer
locoregional therapy, 110
pain management, 79, 82*f*
recurrence of, 110
staging, 108–109
treatment, 109
regorafenib (Stivarga), 3*t*, 100, 108
renal cell carcinoma
bone metastases, 165
chemotherapy, 164
clear cell, 162
epidemiology, 161
genetics of, 162
locoregional therapy, 164–165
papillary, 162
pathology, 161
prognosis, 165
radiation therapy, 164
radiofrequency ablation, 37, 40*f*, 50, 163
staging (TNM), 162–163
surgery, 163
RFA. *see* radiofrequency ablation
rituximab (Rituxan), 2*t*, 100–101
RR, 207

S

sandostatin (octreotide), 98
SD, 207
selective internal radiation therapy (SIRT), 25
SHARP trial, 129
single group trials, 202
SIR-Spheres, 25
SMAD4 mutation, 113
smoking, 144
SOC, 207
sorafenib (Nexavar), 3*t*, 58–59, 101, 129
splanchnic block, 69
stellate ganglion block, 71
stenting, 63–66, 64–66*f*
Stivarga (regorafenib), 3*t*, 100, 108
sunitinib (Sutent), 3*t*, 101, 119, 164
surgical oncology
anatomy, 12
diagnosis, 13–14

education, conferences in, 10
history of, 11–12
multidisciplinary, 12
multimodality therapy, 14–15
prevention, 13–14
principles of, 11–13
staging, 13–14
SVC syndrome, 150
systemic therapy, 1–3

T

Tarceva (erlotinib), 3*t*, 93, 144
targeted therapies, 2, 3*t*
Taxol (paclitaxel), 99
Taxotere (docetaxel), 91, 179
teratogenesis, 27
terminology, 206–207
TheraSphere, 25
thoracentesis/paracentesis, 83–85
topotecan, 102
TP53 mutation, 104, 113, 126, 139
transarterial chemoembolization (TACE)
carcinoid, 124
cholangiocarcinoma, 135
pancreatic neuroendocrine tumor, 119
principles, 51–52, 53*f*, 59, 60*f*
transarterial radioembolization (TARE), 25
transitional cell cancer
chemotherapy, 171
cytologic characteristics, 168
genetics of, 168–169
interventional radiology, 172
locoregional therapy, 171
pathology, 168
prognosis, 169, 171–172
radiation therapy, 171
staging (TNM), 169–170
surgery, 170
transurethral resection of bladder tumor (TURBT), 170
trastuzumab, 2*t*
TSC2 mutation, 117
tuberous sclerosis, 118, 162
tumor ablation, 36–41, 38–40*f*
tumor recurrence, 37, 38–39*f*, 60*f*

tunneled central line (Hickman catheter), 42–43*f*, 42–44, 45–46*f*
tunneled PICC, 47
Turcot's syndrome, 105

U

urothelial cancers
chemotherapy, 171
cytologic characteristics, 168
epidemiology, 168
genetics of, 168–169
interventional radiology, 172
locoregional therapy, 171
prognosis, 169, 171–172
radiation therapy, 171
staging (TNM), 169–170
surgery, 170

V

vaginal cancer, 193–196
Vectibix (panitumumab), 99
veno-occlusive disease, 29, 54–55
venous access devices, 41–44, 42–43*f*, 45–46*f*
vertebral augmentation, 72–76, 74–75*f*, 77*f*
vincristine, 102
vinorelbine (Navelbine), 103
von Hippel–Lindau syndrome, 117, 162
VP-16 (etoposide), 93

W

WNT pathway, 104

X

Xeloda (capecitabine), 90

Y

Yervoy (ipilimumab), 2, 2*t*, 96

Z

Zofran (ondansetron), 98